Renal Diet Cookbook

~100+~

Amazingly Delicious Low Sodium, Potassium and Phosphorus Recipes to Prevent Kidney Disease and Avoid Dialysis

KELSEY CROSS

© Copyright 2020 by KELSEY CROSS- All rights reserved.

This document is geared towards providing exact and reliable information in regard to the topic and issue covered. The publication is sold with the idea that the publisher is not required to render accounting, officially permitted, or otherwise, qualified services. If advice is necessary, legal or professional, a practiced individual in the profession should be ordered.

- From a Declaration of Principles which was accepted and approved equally by a Committee of the American Bar Association and a Committee of Publishers and Associations.

In no way is it legal to reproduce, duplicate, or transmit any part of this document in either electronic means or in printed format. Recording of this publication is strictly prohibited and any storage of this document is not allowed unless with written permission from the publisher. All rights reserved.

The information provided herein is stated to be truthful and consistent, in that any liability, in terms of inattention or otherwise, by any usage or abuse of any policies, processes, or directions contained within is the solitary and utter responsibility of the recipient reader. Under no circumstances will any legal responsibility or blame be held against the publisher for any reparation, damages, or monetary loss due to the information herein, either directly or indirectly.

Respective authors own all copyrights not held by the publisher.

The information herein is offered for informational purposes solely and is universal as so. The presentation of the information is without contract or any type of guarantee assurance.

The trademarks that are used are without any consent, and the publication of the trademark is without permission or backing by the trademark owner. All trademarks and brands within this book are for clarifying purposes only and are owned by the owners themselves, not affiliated with this document.

TABLE OF CONTENTS

INTRODUCTION 6

BREAKFAST 8
    1. Apple and Cinnamon French Toast Strata 8
    2. Apple and Onion Omelet 8
    3. Asparagus and Cauliflower Tortilla 9
    4. Avocado Toast with Egg 10
    5. Baked Egg Cups 11
    6. Breakfast Burrito 12
    7. Chorizo and Egg Tortilla 12
    8. Cottage Cheese Pancakes 13
    9. Egg Cups 13
    10. Breakfast Casserole 14
    11. Grilled Veggie and Cheese Bagel 15

MAINS 16
    12. Curry Chicken 16
    13. Spicy Lamb 16
    14. Special Pizza 17
    15. Slow-Cooked Lemon Chicken 18
    16. Classic Beef Stroganoff with Egg Noodles 19
    17. Roast Pork Loin with Sweet and Tart Apple Stuffing 20
    18. Slow-Cooked Bavarian Pot Roast 22

SIDES 24
    19. Roasted Onion Dip 24
    20. Roasted Garlic White Bean Dip 24
    21. Green Goddess Dip 25
    22. Crab and Carrot Dip 26
    23. Roasted Mint Carrots 26
    24. Roasted Root Vegetables 27
    25. Vegetable Couscous 28

SEAFOOD 29
    26. Lemony Haddock 29
    27. Glazed Salmon 29
    28. Tuna Casserole 30
    29. Oregano Salmon with Crunchy Crust 31
    30. Sardine Fish Cakes 31
    31. Cajun Catfish 32
    32. Poached Gennaro/Sea Bass with Red Peppers 33
    33. Shrimp Skewers with Mango Cucumber Salsa 33

POULTRY 35
    34. Roasted Citrus Chicken 35
    35. Chicken with Asian Vegetables 35
    36. Chicken Adobo 36
    37. Chicken and Veggie Soup 37
    38. Turkey Sausages 38
    39. Rosemary Chicken 38
    40. Smokey Turkey Chili 39
    41. Chicken Kebab Sandwich 40
    42. Aromatic Chicken and Cabbage Stir-Fry 41

MEAT 42

43. Mouthwatering Beef and Chilli Stew 42
44. Beef and Three Pepper Stew 43
45. Sticky Pulled Beef Open Sandwiches 44
46. Herby Beef Stroganoff and Fluffy Rice 45
47. Chunky Beef and Potato Slow Roast 46
48. Chinese-style Beef Stew 47
49. Beef One-Pot Slow Roast 48
50. Pineapple and Mint Lamb Chops 49
51. Spiced Lamb Burgers 49
52. Roast Beef 50
53. Pork Peccadillo 51
54. Chapter 7: Vegetable 51
55. Asparagus and carrot salad with burrata 53
56. Quinoa salad Winning 53
57. Spinach Mango Vegetables 54
58. Braised Swiss chard with garlic and balsamic vinegar 55
59. Snow peas all with thyme 56
60. Cauliflower and fresh dill 56
61. Cauliflower and Potato Curry 57
62. Tofu Stir Fry 58
63. Broccoli Pancake 59
64. Carrot Casserole 60
65. Eggplant Fries 60

SOUPS AND STEWS 62

66. Paprika Pork Soup 62
67. Mediterranean Vegetable Soup 62
68. Tofu Soup 63
69. Beef Stew 64
70. Lamb Stew 65

SNACKS 67

71. Baked Jicama Fries 67
72. Double-Boiled Sweet Potatoes 68
73. Fried Shrimps with Sauce 68
74. Hard-Boiled Eggs with Onions 70
75. Simple Cookies 71
76. Popcorn with Sauce 72
77. Edamame Dip 72
78. Moo-Less Chocolate Mousse 73
79. Baked Carrots 74
80. Cranberry & Apple Coleslaw 74
81. Apple and Fennel Salad 75

DESSERTS 76

82. Lemon Squares 76
83. Homemade apple sauce 77
84. Ice cream sandwiches 77
85. Creamy Pineapple Dessert 78
86. Blackberry Mountain Pie 78
87. Baked Apple Pie 79
88. Whipped Strawberry Mousse 79
89. Chocolate Chips Fudge 80
90. Chocolate Molten Lava Cake 81

91.	Coconut Almond Cake	82
92.	Dark Chocolate Cake	82
93.	Sweet Blueberry Lemon Cake	83
94.	Lemon Coconut Cream Dessert	85
95.	Pumpkin Pie Pudding	85
96.	Sugar-Free Fudge	86
97.	Peppermint Extract Fudge	87
98.	Key Lime Cheesecake	87
99.	Sticky Toffee Pudding	89
100.	Spiced Candied Nuts	90
101.	Chocolate Chip Cookies	91

30-DAY MEAL PLAN 93

CONCLUSION 95

INTRODUCTION

Kidney disease affects millions of people, and is a growing epidemic. Millions are living with chronic kidney disease (CKD), which is an inflammatory disease. An estimated 10% of Americans over the age of fifty have kidney disease of which the majority is not even aware of. For many, the disease progresses until their kidneys stop functioning. As a result, people with chronic kidney disease must undergo dialysis or dialysis along with a kidney transplant.

In the United States, African Americans, Mexican Americans and Native Americans are disproportionately affected by kidney disease i.e. African Americans are three times as likely as Caucasians to develop kidney disease before the age of 60. 1 In the United States, 20 percent of African Americans have been diagnosed with chronic kidney disease (CKD), which is the failure of kidney function. This rate is four times higher than the one of Caucasians. For Mexican Americans, an increase of 3.9 times higher is reported. The prevalence of vitamin D deficiency is twice as high in Hispanic Americans as in Caucasians. Vitamin D deficiency may be linked to kidney disease. Many hypotheses have been raised regarding the etiology of chronic kidney disease (CKD).

Chronic kidney disease affects millions of people around the world and until now no effective drugs have been discovered that can quickly cure it, prevent it or slow down its progression. A recent study has found a link between chronic kidney disease and vitamin D deficiency and the possible role of vitamin D in protecting against CKD.

Vitamin D is a secosteroid hormone precursor that is important for bones, muscles and immune functions. Vitamin D deficiency is prevalent in most populations around the world and in African Americans and Mexican Americans is even higher than Caucasians.

Chronic kidney disease is associated with reduced bone mass that can lead to osteoporosis and loss of muscle mass and function. It is also associated with increased risk of cardiovascular disease and higher mortality in the general population. CKD is also linked with increased risk of osteomalacia which is characterized by decreased bone mineral density and muscle weakness.

Kidney function includes filtration, absorption and secretion of various substances. That is why kidney health is important for an individual's overall health and well-being. An impaired kidney function can affect the performance of the central nervous system and can also lead to loss of appetite and strength in general. A decreased kidney function is also associated with hyperparathyroidism (hyperplasia of parathyroid glands, which can lead to renal osteodystrophy and renal osteopenia and deterioration of kidneys) which may in turn lead to kidney failure.

Renal diet for people with chronic kidney disease includes a low phosphorus, low potassium and low sodium meals. The renal diet should include a meal plan high in fruits, vegetables, grains, and lean protein. It is also famous for high quantities of fluids and water but is devoid of salt (sodium) and phosphorus. The renal diet also states that a person should avoid animal proteins and fats. But fruits and vegetables that are rich in calcium, antioxidants and fiber are to be included in the diet.

Renal diet for people with chronic kidney disease is a very important aspect of nutritional therapy recommended by kidney diet physicians.

It is recommended to create a plan with a nephrologist and let them monitor the trends and changes of kidney function. It is also crucial to have a good dietary plan. Remember that food can be very healing. In this way we can prevent many complications and fight the inflammation.

This renal diet cookbook will help you learn how to prepare delicious meals that are helpful for patients suffering from chronic kidney disease. These meal suggestions have been designed by doctors who specialize in CKD management. For healthy people, renal diets may seem too restrictive or boring, but for people with any kind of kidney disease, this kind of diet is the key to improving kidney function, slowing down the progression of the disease and ultimately preventing kidney failure. To better control what you eat and reduce what doesn't work for your kidneys you should cook more at home. Yes, it's that simple as 80% of sodium intake comes from processed food. If you cook at home you have a better view on the sodium, phosphorus and potassium quantity. With the recipes that we have prepared you can easily adapt to using and needing it less.

We can always be proactive in our health and choices around kidney disease. It's not about the past but about how we manage our health in the future.

BREAKFAST

1. Apple and Cinnamon French Toast Strata

Preparation Time: 2 Hours and 20 Minutes

Cooking Time: 50 Minutes

Servings: 12

INGREDIENTS:

- 1 ½ medium apples peeled, cored, diced
- 1-pound cinnamon and raisin loaf, diced
- 1 teaspoon ground cinnamon
- ¼ cup pancake syrup
- 6 tablespoons unsalted butter, melted
- 1 ¼ cup half-and-half creamer
- 8 ounces cream cheese, softened and cubed
- 8 large eggs
- 1 ¼ cup almond milk, unsweetened

DIRECTIONS:

1. Take a 9 by 13 inches baking dish, grease it with oil, then arrange half of the bread cubes on the bottom and scatter cream cheese evenly on the top.
2. Top cream cheese with the apple, sprinkle with cinnamon, and then top with remaining bread cubes.
3. Crack eggs in a large bowl, add pancake syrup, butter, milk, and creamer, whisk until combined, pour this mixture evenly in the prepared casserole, cover it with plastic wrap, and then keep the casserole dish in the refrigerator for 2 hours.
4. When ready to cook, switch on the oven, then set it to 325°F, and let it preheat.
5. Then uncover the casserole, bake for 50 minutes. When done, let it cool for 10 minutes and cut it into twelve 3 by 3-inches squares.
6. Drizzle with more pancake syrup and then serve.

NUTRITION: Calories 324, Fat 20 g, Protein 9 g, Carbohydrates 27 g, Fiber 1.8 g

2. Apple and Onion Omelet

Preparation Time: 10 Minutes

Cooking Time: 20 Minutes

Servings: 2

INGREDIENTS:

- 1 large apple peeled, cored, sliced
- ¾ cup sweet onion, sliced
- 1 tablespoon unsalted butter
- 1/8 teaspoon ground black pepper
- 1 tablespoon water
- ¼ cup milk, low-fat
- 2 tablespoons shredded cheddar cheese, low-fat
- 3 eggs

DIRECTIONS:

1. Switch on the oven, then set it to 400°F and let it preheat.
2. Crack eggs in a bowl, add black pepper and water, and whisk until beaten.
3. Take a small heat proof skillet pan, place it over medium heat, add butter and when it melts, add onions and apple, and cook for 6 minutes until sauteed.
4. Spread onion-apple mixture evenly, pour egg mixture over it, spread evenly, and cook for 2 minutes until eggs begin to set.
5. Then sprinkle cheese on top of eggs, transfer skillet pan into the heated oven, and bake for 12 minutes or until the omelet has set.
6. When done, remove the pan from the oven, cut the omelet in half, distribute it between two plates, and then serve.

NUTRITION: Calories 282, Fat 16 g, Protein 13 g, Carbohydrates 22 g, Fiber 3.5 g

3. Asparagus and Cauliflower Tortilla

Preparation Time: 10 Minutes

Cooking Time: 25 Minutes

Servings: 4

INGREDIENTS:

- 2 cups asparagus, chopped and trimmed
- 1 ½ cups white onion, chopped
- 2 cups cauliflower florets, chopped
- ½ teaspoon minced garlic
- ¼ teaspoon ground nutmeg

- ½ teaspoon ground black pepper
- ¼ teaspoon salt
- ¼ teaspoon dried thyme leaves
- 2 tablespoons parsley, chopped
- 2 teaspoons olive oil
- 1 cup liquid egg substitute, low cholesterol
- 1 tablespoon water

DIRECTIONS:

1. Take a heatproof bowl, add cauliflower florets and asparagus, drizzle with water, cover the bowl with plastic wrap, pierce some holes in it, and microwave for 5 minutes, or until tender-crisp.
2. Meanwhile, take a medium-sized skillet pan, place it over medium heat, add oil, and when hot, add onion and cook for 7 minutes until golden brown.
3. Stir in garlic, cook for 1 minute until fragrant, switch heat to medium-low level, add steamed cauliflower-asparagus mixture in the pan, sprinkle with nutmeg, black pepper, salt, thyme, and parsley, and pour in egg substitute.
4. Continue cooking for 10 to 15 minutes, or until the tortilla has set and the bottom is nicely browned, and when done, slide the tortilla onto a dish by running the knife along the edges.
5. Cut the tortilla into four pieces and then serve.

NUTRITION: Calories 102, Fat 3 g, Protein 9 g, Carbohydrates 9 g, Fiber 3.8 g

4. Avocado Toast with Egg

Preparation Time: 10 Minutes

Cooking Time: 5 Minutes

Servings: 2 Toasts

INGREDIENTS:

- ½ of a medium avocado, pitted and sliced
- 1 tablespoon parsley, chopped
- ¼ teaspoon ground black pepper
- 1/8 teaspoon salt
- 1 tablespoon lime juice
- 2 tablespoons feta cheese, crumbled
- 2 eggs

- 2 slices of whole-grain bread, toasted

DIRECTIONS:

1. Transfer avocado flesh to a medium bowl, mash with a fork, and then stir in salt and lime juice.
2. Spread the avocado mixture evenly onto each piece of toast, then take a skillet pan, spray it with oil and when hot, crack eggs into it and cook to the desired level.
3. Distribute eggs onto the toast, top each piece of toast with ½ tablespoon parsley, 1 tablespoon cheese, and 1/8 teaspoon ground black pepper.
4. Serve straight away.

NUTRITION: Calories 225, Fat 13 g, Protein 12 g, Carbohydrates 15g, Fiber 4.3 g

5. Baked Egg Cups

Preparation Time: 20 Minutes

Cooking Time: 35 Minutes

Servings: 12 Muffins

INGREDIENTS:

- 1/3 cup mushrooms, diced
- ¼ teaspoon ground black pepper
- 1/3 cup green bell pepper, diced
- 1/3 cup white onion, diced
- 6 slices bacon, low sodium
- 12 eggs

DIRECTIONS:

1. Switch on the oven, then set it to 350°F and let it preheat.
2. Meanwhile, take a twelve-cup muffin tray, line it with muffin liners, and set aside until required.
3. Take a medium-sized skillet pan, place it over medium heat and when hot, add bacon slices and cook for 7 to 10 minutes, or until crispy.
4. When the bacon has cooked, transfer it to a cutting board, let it cool for 5 minutes, chop the bacon, and then transfer it to a bowl.
5. Add all the vegetables in the bowl containing bacon, stir until well mixed, and then distribute the mixture evenly between prepared muffin cups.
6. Take another bowl, crack eggs in it, add black pepper, whisk until combined, pour this mixture evenly into muffin cups, and bake into the heated oven for 25 minutes, or until firm and when the tops are golden brown.

7. When done, let muffins cool for 5 minutes, then take them out, let the muffins cool for an additional 10 minutes, and serve.

NUTRITION: Calories 80, Fat 5 g, Protein 7 g, Carbohydrates 1 g, Fiber – 0.1 g

6. Breakfast Burrito

Preparation Time: 10 Minutes

Cooking Time: 3 Minutes

Servings: 2

INGREDIENTS:

- 3 tablespoons green chiles, diced
- ½ teaspoon hot pepper sauce
- ¼ teaspoon ground cumin
- 4 eggs
- 2 flour tortillas, burrito size

DIRECTIONS:

1. Take a medium-sized skillet pan, place it over medium heat, grease it with oil, and let it get hot.
2. Crack eggs in a bowl, add chilies, hot sauce, and cumin, whisk until combined, then pour the egg mixture in the hot skillet and cook for 2 minutes, or until eggs have been cooked to the desired level.
3. Meanwhile, heat the tortillas by microwaving them for 20 seconds until hot.
4. When eggs have cooked, distribute evenly between hot tortillas, and roll it up like a burrito.
5. Serve straight away.

NUTRITION: Calories 366, Fat 18 g, Protein 18 g, Carbohydrates 33 g, Fiber 2.5 g

7. Chorizo and Egg Tortilla

Preparation Time: 10 Minutes

Cooking Time: 13 Minutes

Servings: 1

INGREDIENTS:

- 1 flour tortilla, about 6-inches
- 1/3 cup Chorizo meat, chopped
- 1 egg

DIRECTIONS:

1. Take a medium-sized skillet pan, place it over medium heat and when hot, add Chorizo and cook for 5 to 8 minutes until done.
2. When the meat has cooked, drain the excess fat, whisk an egg, pour it into the pan, stir until combined, and cook for 3 minutes, or until eggs have cooked.
3. Spoon egg onto the tortilla, and then serve.

NUTRITION: Calories 223, Fat 11 g, Protein 16 g, Carbohydrates 15 g, Fiber 1.5 g

8. Cottage Cheese Pancakes

Preparation Time: 10 Minutes

Cooking Time: 50 Minutes

Servings: 6

INGREDIENTS:

- 3 cups fresh raspberries, sliced
- ½ cup all-purpose white flour
- 1 cup cottage cheese, softened
- 6 tablespoons unsalted butter, melted
- 4 eggs, beaten

DIRECTIONS:

1. Crack eggs in a medium-sized bowl, add flour, cheese, and butter in it, and whisk until combined.
2. Take a medium-high frying pan, grease it with oil and when hot, pour in prepared batter, ¼ cup of batter per pancake, spread the batter into a 4-inch pancake, and cook for 3 minutes per side until browned.
3. When done, transfer pancakes onto a plate, cook more pancakes in the same manner, and, when done, serve each pancake with ½ sliced raspberries.

NUTRITION: Calories 253, Fat 17 g, Protein 11 g, Carbohydrates 21 g, Fiber – 2 g

9. Egg Cups

Preparation Time: 10 minutes

Cooking Time: 30 minutes

Servings: 12

INGREDIENTS:

- ¼ cup Shiitake mushrooms—diced

- 1/3 cup bell peppers—diced
- 1/3 cup onion—diced
- 12 eggs
- ½ teaspoon oregano—dried or fresh

DIRECTIONS:

1. As you are cutting and washing vegetables and mushrooms, make sure that your oven is preheated to 350 degrees F° and that your baking dish is ready. You can place a tin foil over the baking dish and arrange 12 muffin cups.
2. The next step is to take a bowl and beat the eggs, and add oregano. Let the eggs rest while you take care of the veggies and mushrooms. Take a frying pan or any kind of cooking dish, add some olive oil, not more than a tablespoon, and saute the onion. After several minutes of sauteing and stirring, add peppers and mushrooms to the pan and saute some more until the veggies are mildly softened, and the onion is slightly browned. Add the veggie mixture to the bowl with eggs, combine it all well with a spoon then fill muffin cups with the mixture you have prepared. Place the baking dish into the oven and bake for 25 minutes.

NUTRITION: Potassium 90mg, Sodium 70mg, Phosphorus 100mg, Calories: 80mg

10. Breakfast Casserole

Preparation time: 10 minutes

Cooking time: 60 minutes

Servings: 8

INGREDIENTS:

- 200 grams of lean ground beef—fresh and grass-fed if possible
- ½ cup cream cheese
- 4 slices of bread white, cut in cubes
- 5 eggs
- 1 teaspoon of mustard—dry
- ½ teaspoon garlic powder with no added sodium

DIRECTIONS:

1. Preheat your oven to 350 degrees F as you are preparing ingredients for the breakfast casserole. Cube bread sliced and place it aside while you are taking care of the ground beef.
2. As you prepare the beef, add a tablespoon of olive oil to the skillet and add the beef. Cook the beef with occasional stirring as you are breaking the meat parts to bits.
3. Once the meat is browned, set aside and add garlic powder, stirring it well to combine. Beat the five eggs

in a bowl, then combine all ingredients in the egg bowl, and mix to get a homogenous mass out of the egg mixture.

4. Pour the mixture into the mildly greased baking dish and place it in the oven
5. Bake for 50 minutes or until ready.

NUTRITION: Potassium 176mg, Sodium 201mg, Phosphorus 119mg, Calories 220

11. Grilled Veggie and Cheese Bagel

Preparation time: 10 minutes

Cooking time: 5 minutes

Servings: 1

INGREDIENTS:

- 1 white flour bagel—sliced in half
- ½ cup arugula
- ½ cup low-sodium cheese or cream cheese (lower potassium, higher sodium)
- ¼ red onion—finely sliced
- 2 slices eggplant—roasted or grilled
- ½ teaspoon lemon pepper

DIRECTIONS:

1. First, you need to deal with preparing veggies and slicing, and once the preparation is finished, grill 2 slices of eggplant with some lemon pepper spread over the slices.
2. Baking the eggplant slices would be another option in case you don't have an option to grill the slices.
3. You may roast the eggplant by placing it on a tin foil or a baking paper set on a baking dish in a preheated oven for 5 minutes each side of the slices.
4. Once the eggplant is grilled, toast the bagel sliced in two as for making a sandwich the same way the eggplant was grilled, but reduced to grilling each side 2 minutes or less.
5. Spread some cheese on the bagel, add the eggplant slices and the rest of the ingredients.
6. Seal the bagel with the top part, and you have a great start to the day.

NUTRITION: Potassium 112mg, Sodium 186mg, Phosphorus 50mg, Calories 114

MAINS

12. Curry Chicken

Preparation Time: 10 minutes

Cooking Time: 45 minutes

Servings: 6 portions

INGREDIENTS:

- Chicken, 1 whole, cut in small parts, skin removed
- Lemon juice, ¼ cup
- Dry thyme, ½ tsp
- Curry powder, 2 tsp
- Onion, 1 medium, chopped
- Garlic clove, 1 medium chopped (optional)
- Black pepper, ½ tsp
- Vegetable, 2 tbsp. (or olive oil)
- Water, 1 cup

DIRECTIONS:

1. Pour lemon juice on cleaned Chicken and wash it.
2. Combine seasoning together in a bowl and rub it on chicken parts.
3. Marinate the seasoned chicken overnight in the refrigerator (can be used after 1 hour).
4. In a saucepan, heat oil, fry seasoned Chicken until browned.
5. From the marinated bowl, Rinse remaining seasoning with water.
6. Pour this remaining marinade over browned Chicken. Let cook on low heat until tender.
7. Place over hot rice and serve.

NUTRITION: Calories 21 gr, Protein 24 gr, Total Fat 5 gr, Carbohydrate 93 mg, Sodium 317 mg, Potassium 214 mg, Phosphorus

13. Spicy Lamb

Preparation Time: 20 minutes

Cooking Time: 1 hour and 30 minutes

Servings: 4 portions

INGREDIENTS:

- 1 lamb leg (trimmed for roasting)
- Vegetable oil, ¼ cup
- Garlic powder, 1 ½ tbsp.
- Dry mustard, 3 tsp

DIRECTIONS:

1. Mix ingredients for the marinade: garlic powder, oil, and mustard.
2. Rub leg of lamb with marinade thoroughly; refrigerate overnight or for 6-8 hours.
3. Heat barbecue spit Adjust meat on it and bake drizzling meat constantly with marinade until,
4. 170°F on a meat thermometer or for 30 minutes per pound.

NUTRITION: 289 Calories, 24g Protein, 6g total Fat, 3g Carbohydrate, 144 mg Sodium, 423 mg Potassium, 237 mg, Phosphorus

14. Special Pizza

Preparation Time: 25 minutes

Cooking Time: 15 minutes

Servings: 10 slices

INGREDIENTS FOR CRUST:

- Active dry yeast, 1 tsp
- Granulated sugar, 1 tbsp.
- Water, 1 cup
- All-purpose flour, 2 cups
- Vegetable shortening, 2 tbsp.

DIRECTIONS:

1. In a mixing bowl, mix flour, sugar, and yeast.
2. Add in shortening to the above ingredients; mix all together using a fork.
3. Include water in little quantities while mixing together with the fork until the mixture combines well together and follows the fork around the bowl.
4. Allow the dough to rest after covering for about 15 minutes.

INGREDIENTS FOR PIZZA:

- Ground beef, ½ pound lean (or Chicken or turkey)
- Italian seasoning, ½ tsp

- Tomato paste, ¼ cup
- Onion powder, ½ tsp
- Chili powder, 1 tsp
- Garlic powder, ½ tsp
- Italian seasoning, 1 tsp
- Water vegetable oil, ½ cup
- Sharp cheddar cheese, 4 oz. reduced-fat, grated
- Green peppers, ½ cup, diced
- Onions, ½ cup, diced

DIRECTIONS:

1. Heat oven to 425°f.
2. Saute ground meat in a frying pan. Add onion powder, Italian seasoning, and garlic
3. powder; stir continuously until meat is brown.
4. Drain the oil by Placing meat onto paper towels.
5. In a small bowl, prepare the pizza sauce by blending the tomato paste, Italian seasoning, chili powder, and water. Put aside.
6. Take out the rested dough, grease fingers, and pizza pan. Stretch dough on the pan evenly.
7. Evenly Pour sauce over pizza dough; scatter with ½ cup of cheese.
8. Bake in the heated oven for around 15-20 minutes.
9. Take out from the oven; include ground beef, onions, green peppers, and remaining cheese.
10. 1 Put back in the oven for an added 10 minutes. Serve hot.

NUTRITION: 196 Calories, 11g Protein, 7g total Fat, 24g Carbohydrate 144 mg Sodium, 188 mg Potassium, 31 mg Phosphorus

15. Slow-Cooked Lemon Chicken

Preparation Time: 20 minutes

Cooking Time: 5-1/4 hours

Servings: 4

INGREDIENTS

- Dried oregano, 1 tsp
- Ground black pepper, ¼ tsp
- Butter, unsalted, 2 tbsps.

- Chicken breast, 1 pound, boneless, skinless
- Chicken broth, ¼ cup, low sodium
- Water, ¼ cup
- Lemon juice, 1 tbsp.
- Garlic, minced, 2 cloves
- Fresh basil, 1 tsp, chopped

DIRECTIONS:

1. In a small bowl, mix oregano and grounded black pepper. Coat mixture on the chicken.
2. In a medium skillet, soften the butter over medium heat. Cook the chicken in the melted butter till it is golden brown and then shift the chicken to the slow cooker.
3. To loosen the brown bits stuck in the skillet, pour water, chicken broth, garlic, and lemon juice in the skillet, get it to a boil. Pour this over the browned chicken.
4. Close the slow cooker and set on low for 5 hours or on high for 2½ hours.
5. Baste chicken and Add basil. For an additional 15–30 minutes, Cover and cook on high or until chicken is soft and tender.

NUTRITION: 197 Calorie, 26g Protein, 9g Total Fat, 1g Carbohydrates 57 mg Sodium, 251 mg Phosphorus, 412 mg Potassium

16. Classic Beef Stroganoff with Egg Noodles

Preparation Time: 15 minutes

Cooking Time: 15 minutes

Servings:6

INGREDIENTS

- Onions, 1 cup, finely diced
- Egg, beaten, 1
- Worcestershire sauce, 2 tbsp., reduced-sodium
- Breadcrumbs, ¼ cup
- Mayonnaise, 1 tbsp.
- Tomato sauce, 1 tbsp., no salt added
- Ground beef, 1 pound
- Canola oil, 3 tbsp.
- Flour, 2 tbsp.

- Water, 3 cups
- Black pepper, 1 tsp, freshly ground
- Better than bouillon beef, 4 tsp, reduced-sodium
- Sour cream, ¼ cup
- 2 tbsp. chives
- Wide egg noodles, ½ package (12oz package), cooked
- Butter, unsalted, 2 tbsp., cold and cubed
- Parsley, ¼ cup
- Rosemary, chopped, 1 tbsp.

DIRECTIONS:

1. Mix the first six ingredients and half tsp black pepper in a big bowl. Add in the ground beef and mix thoroughly. Make 16 meatballs of the same size.
2. Cook Stroganoff meatballs in a big fry pan until browned on medium heat. Shift all meatballs to one area and add oil and flour to the same pan and stir until well-combined. Add the remaining black pepper, water, and bouillon, and then keep stirring until sauce thickens, for 10 minutes.
3. Take off the heat and mix in chives and sour cream, then serve over egg noodles.
4. Pasta:
5. To a large pan, add egg noodles with 2 tbsp. of water, heat and mix until warm, then take off the heat. Mix in butter, rosemary, and parsley until everything is well incorporated.

NUTRITION: 490 Calories, 20gr Protein, 32g Total Fat, 30g Carbohydrates 598 mg Sodium, 230 mg Phosphorus 230, 423 mg Potassium

17. Roast Pork Loin with Sweet and Tart Apple Stuffing

Preparation Time: 45 minutes

Cooking Time: 1 hour

Servings: 6

INGREDIENTS:

- Cherry marmalade glaze:
- Dried cherries, ¼ cup
- Orange marmalade, ½ cup sugar-free
- Nutmeg, 1/8 tsp
- Apple juice, ¼ cup

- Cinnamon, 1/8 tsp
- Apple stuffing:
- Canola oil, 2 tbsp.
- Hawaiian rolls, 2 cups packed cubed (or any white bread)
- Granny smith, ½ cup, finely diced (honey crisp or Macintosh apple)
- Butter, 2 tbsp., unsalted
- Onions, finely diced, 2 tbsp.
- Celery, finely diced, 2 tbsp.
- Fresh thyme, 1 tbsp., (or dried thyme, ½ tsp)
- Black pepper, 1 tsp
- Chicken stock, low-sodium, ½ cup
- Roast pork loin:
- Pork loin, 1 pound, boneless
- Butcher twine, two 18-inch pieces

DIRECTIONS:

1. Glaze Cherry Marmalade:
2. In a small pan, mix all the glaze ingredients on medium-high heat till marmalade is liquefied and starts to bubble. Take off heat and put aside.
3. Heat oven to 400° F.
4. Apple Stuffing:
5. In a large sauté pan, slightly fry all ingredients in oil on medium-high heat for 2–3 minutes except for chicken stock.
6. Gradually add chicken stock until moist, but not too wet. (may not be needed as it may depend on how much juice is released from the apples during cooking.)
7. Take off from heat and cool it to room temperature.
8. Pork Loin:
9. In the meantime, form several pockets by cutting five slits along the length of the loin, about 1 inch apart
10. Fill each pocket with around 2 tbsp. of stuffing (saving around a half cup)
11. To keep the stuffing in place, tie the twine around the loin as needed.
12. Put the remaining stuffing on a baking tray, top with tied stuffed pork, and bake for 45 minutes at 400° F, check with an internal temperature should be 160° F.
13. 1 Glaze with the prepared dried cherry marmalade, turn off the oven and let the loin rest inside the oven

for 10–15 minutes. Take out a pork loin, slice into portions and enjoy the meal.

NUTRITION: 263 Calories, 22g Carbohydrates, 14g Protein, 14g Fat, 137 mg Sodium, 154 mg Phosphorus, 275 mg Potassium

18. Slow-Cooked Bavarian Pot Roast

Preparation Time: 15 minutes

Cooking Time: 8 hours

Servings: 12

INGREDIENTS:

- Beef chuck roast, 3 pounds
- Vegetable oil, 1 tsp
- Ginger, ½ tsp, freshly ground
- Pepper, ½ tsp
- Cloves, 3, whole
- Apples, 2 cups, sliced
- Onions, ½ cup, sliced
- Apple juice, ½ cup (or water)
- Flour, 4 tbsp.
- 4 tbsp. water
- Fresh apple slices, optional garnish

DIRECTIONS:

1. Trim the extra fat from the beef roast. Wash and dry with a napkin. Rub the roast's top with oil, then scatter with ginger and pepper and add the whole cloves to the whole roast. Next, in a hot pan greased with oil, sear both sides of the pot roast.
2. In a crock-pot or a slow cooker, place the onions and apples. Place the pot roast and splash the roast with apple juice.
3. Cook on low heat covered for 10 to 12 hours, or around 5-6 hours, on high.
4. Extract the roast from the slow cooker. Put it aside; keep it warm, though.
5. Drain the juices from the pot roast and funnel them straight into the slow cooker. To reduce this liquid and thicken it, turn the heat to high.
6. Using flour and water, make a nice paste, then pour into the slow cooker, whisking as you mix.
7. Cover and boil until the mixture thickens. Just prior to serving, pour over the roast.
8. Optional: Garnish with slices of fresh apples.

NUTRITION: 313 Calories, 6g Carbohydrates, 22g Protein, 22g Total Fat, 73 mg Sodium, 2020 mg Phosphorus, 373 mg Potassium

SIDES

19. Roasted Onion Dip

Preparation Time: 15 minutes

Cooking Time: 35 minutes

Servings: 1½ cups

INGREDIENTS:

- 1 red onion, chopped
- 2 tablespoons extra-virgin olive oil
- 1 (8-ounce) package cream cheese, at room temperature
- 2 tablespoons mayonnaise (made with avocado oil or olive oil)
- 1 tablespoon freshly squeezed lemon juice
- ½ teaspoon dried thyme leaves

DIRECTIONS:

1. Preheat the oven to 400°F.
2. On a rimmed baking sheet, combine the onion and olive oil and toss to coat.
3. Roast for 30 to 35 minutes, stirring occasionally, until the onions are soft and golden brown. Don't let them burn. Transfer to a plate and set aside.
4. In a medium bowl, beat the cream cheese, mayonnaise, lemon juice, and thyme leaves. Stir in the onions.
5. You can serve the dip at this point or cover and refrigerate it up to 8 hours before serving.
6. Appliance Tip: You can roast onions in a slow cooker in larger quantities for bulk cooking or if you're throwing a party. Place 4 to 5 chopped onions and ¼ cup of olive oil in a 3-quart slow cooker. Cover and cook on low for 7 to 9 hours or until the onions are golden brown and tender. You can freeze the onions in ½-cup portions and add to soups, casseroles, side dishes, or stews.

NUTRITION: Per Serving (3 tablespoons) Calories: 212; Total fat: 21g; Saturated fat: 9g; Sodium: 149mg; Phosphorus: 47mg; Potassium: 82mg; Carbohydrates: 4g; Fiber: 0g; Protein: 3g; Sugar: 2g

20. Roasted Garlic White Bean Dip

Preparation Time: 20 Minutes

Cooking Time: 60 Minutes

Servings: 2

INGREDIENTS:

- 2 onions, cut into 8 wedges each

- 2 garlic heads, whole
- ¼ cup extra-virgin olive oil, divided
- 1 (15-ounce) can no-salt-added cannellini beans, drained and rinsed
- 2 tablespoons freshly squeezed lemon juice
- 1 teaspoon dried marjoram leaves
- ⅛ teaspoon salt
- ⅛ teaspoon freshly ground black pepper

DIRECTIONS:

1. Preheat the oven to 375°F.
2. On a rimmed baking sheet, place the onions.
3. Cut the top inch off each garlic head, just enough to expose the cloves, and discard the top. Place the garlic, with the exposed cloves facing up, on the baking sheet. Drizzle 1 tablespoon of olive oil directly into the garlic heads, then wrap each head in aluminum foil and place back on the baking sheet. Drizzle the onions with another 1 tablespoon of olive oil.
4. Roast the vegetables for 45 to 55 minutes, stirring the onions once during cooking, until the onions are golden brown, and the garlic is brown and soft.
5. Remove the foil from the garlic and let the garlic and onions cool for 30 minutes.
6. In a blender or food processor, combine the cannellini beans, lemon juice, marjoram, salt, and pepper.
7. Add the onions. Remove the garlic cloves from the head by squeezing the head so the cloves pop out and add to the blender. Blend or process the mixture, drizzling in the remaining 2 tablespoons of olive oil, until it is mostly smooth, with some texture.
8. Serve immediately or cover and chill for a few hours before serving.

NUTRITION: Calories 166, Total fat 10g, Saturated fat 1g, Sodium 74mg, Phosphorus 81mg, Potassium 241mg, Carbohydrates 17g, Fiber 4g, Protein 4g, Sugar 2g

21. Green Goddess Dip

Preparation Time: 15 Minutes

Cooking Time: 0 Minutes

Servings: 1 ½ cups

INGREDIENTS:

- 1 (8-ounce) package cream cheese, at room temperature
- 3 tablespoons freshly squeezed lemon juice
- 2 teaspoons Worcestershire sauce

- ½ cup chopped flat-leaf parsley
- ¼ cup minced fresh chives

DIRECTIONS:

1. In a medium bowl, combine the cream cheese, lemon juice, and Worcestershire sauce and beat until smooth.
2. Stir in the parsley and chives. You can serve the dip immediately or cover and chill for 4 to 6 hours before serving.

NUTRITION: Calories 139, Total fat 13g, Saturated fat 8g, Sodium 147mg, Phosphorus 47mg, Potassium 111mg, Carbohydrates 4g, Fiber 0g, Protein 3g, Sugar 2g

22. Crab and Carrot Dip

Preparation Time: 20 Minutes

Cooking Time: 0 Minutes

Servings: 1 ½ cups

INGREDIENTS:

- 1 cup mascarpone cheese
- 2 tablespoons freshly squeezed lemon juice
- ½ cup lump crab meat, drained
- 1 cup grated carrots
- 4 scallions, both green and white parts, chopped

DIRECTIONS:

1. In a medium bowl, beat the mascarpone and lemon juice until smooth.
2. Look over the crab, removing any bits of cartilage and discarding.
3. Stir the crab, carrots, and scallions into the mascarpone mixture. Serve immediately or cover and chill for 4 to 6 hours before serving.

NUTRITION: Calories 194, Total fat 18g, Saturated fat 11g, Sodium 146mg, Phosphorus 89mg, Potassium 184mg, Carbohydrates 4g, Fiber 1g, Protein 5g, Sugar 3g

23. Roasted Mint Carrots

Preparation Time: 5 minutes

Cooking Time: 20 minutes

Servings: 6

INGREDIENTS:

- 1 pound carrots, trimmed
- 1 tablespoon extra-virgin olive oil
- Freshly ground black pepper
- ¼ cup thinly sliced mint

DIRECTIONS:

1. Preheat the oven to 425°F.
2. Arrange the carrots in a single layer on a rimmed baking sheet. Drizzle with the olive oil, and shake the carrots on the sheet to coat. Season with pepper.
3. Roast for 20 minutes, or until tender and browned, stirring twice while cooking. Sprinkle with the mint and serve.
4. Substitution tip: To lower the potassium in this dish, use 8 ounces of carrots and 8 ounces of turnips cut into cubes. This will cut the potassium to 193mg.

NUTRITION: Per Serving Calories: 51; Total Fat: 2g; Saturated Fat: 0g; Cholesterol: 0mg; Carbohydrates: 7g; Fiber: 2g; Protein: 1g; Phosphorus: 26mg; Potassium: 242mg; Sodium: 52mg

24. Roasted Root Vegetables

Preparation Time: 10 minutes

Cooking Time: 25 minutes

Servings: 6

INGREDIENTS:

- 1 cup chopped turnips
- 1 cup chopped rutabaga
- 1 cup chopped parsnips
- 1 tablespoon extra-virgin olive oil
- 1 teaspoon fresh chopped rosemary
- Freshly ground black pepper

DIRECTIONS:

1. Preheat the oven to 400°F.
2. In a large bowl, toss the turnips, rutabaga, and parsnips with the olive oil and rosemary. Arrange in a single layer on a baking sheet, and season with pepper.
3. Bake until the vegetables are tender and browned, 20 to 25 minutes, stirring once.
4. Substitution tip: Experiment with other fresh herbs in this dish to suit your own tastes. Thyme, tarragon,

oregano, and minced garlic all add unique flavors to these root vegetables.

NUTRITION: Per Serving Calories: 52; Total Fat: 2g; Saturated Fat: 0g; Cholesterol: 0mg; Carbohydrates: 7g; Fiber: 2g; Protein: 1g; Phosphorus: 35mg; Potassium: 205mg; Sodium: 22mg

25. Vegetable Couscous

Preparation Time: 10 minutes

Cooking Time: 15 minutes

Servings: 6

INGREDIENTS:

- 1 tablespoon extra-virgin olive oil
- ½ sweet onion, diced
- 1 carrot, diced
- 1 celery stalk, diced
- ½ cup diced red or yellow bell pepper
- 1 small zucchini, diced
- 1 cup couscous
- 1½ cups Simple Chicken Broth or low-sodium store-bought chicken stock
- ½ teaspoon garlic powder
- Freshly ground black pepper

DIRECTIONS:

1. In a large skillet, heat the olive oil over medium heat. Add the onion, carrot, celery, and bell pepper, and cook, stirring occasionally, until the vegetables are just becoming tender, about 5 to 7 minutes.
2. Add the zucchini, couscous, broth, and garlic powder. Stir to blend, and bring to a boil. Cover and remove from the heat. Let stand for 5 to 8 minutes. Fluff with a fork, season with pepper, and serve.
3. Substitution tip: Swap out vegetables to make this couscous your own creation. Yellow summer squash or patty pan squash can be substituted for the zucchini. Other vegetables, like asparagus, broccoli, or cauliflower, can be added instead of carrots and bell peppers.

NUTRITION: Per Serving Calories: 154; Total Fat: 3g; Saturated Fat: 1g; Cholesterol: 0mg; Carbohydrates: 27g; Fiber: 2g; Protein: 5g; Phosphorus: 83mg; Potassium: 197mg; Sodium: 36mgsides

SEAFOOD

26. Lemony Haddock

Preparation Time: 10 minutes

Cooking Time: 20 minutes

Serving: 1

INGREDIENTS:

- 1 tablespoon melted unsalted butter
- 12-ounces haddock fillets, deboned and skinned
- ½ cup breadcrumbs
- 3 tablespoons chopped fresh parsley
- 1 tablespoon lemon zest
- 1 teaspoon chopped fresh thyme
- ¼ teaspoon black pepper (ground)

DIRECTIONS:

1. Preheat the oven to 350°F.
2. In a mixing bowl, add breadcrumbs, parsley, lemon zest, thyme, and pepper. Combine to mix well.
3. Add butter and combine until you get crumbles.
4. Take a baking sheet and place haddock on it. Add crumb mixture on top.
5. Bake for 18-20 minutes until evenly brown from top.
6. Serve warm.

NUTRITION: Calories: 183; Fat: 4g; Phosphorus: 233mg; Potassium: 305mg; Sodium: 316mg; Carbohydrates: 9g; Protein: 16g.

27. Glazed Salmon

Preparation Time: 10 minutes

Cooking Time: 10 minutes

Serving: 1

INGREDIENTS:

- 4 (3-ounce) salmon fillets
- 1 tablespoon olive oil
- 2 tablespoons honey

- 1 teaspoon lemon zest
- ½ teaspoon Black pepper (ground), to taste
- ½ scallion, chopped

DIRECTIONS:

1. Pat dry salmon with paper towels.
2. In a mixing bowl, add honey, lemon zest, and pepper. Combine to mix well.
3. Add salmon and coat evenly.
4. Take a medium saucepan or skillet, add oil. Heat over medium heat.
5. Add salmon and stir-cook until light brown and cooked well, for about 8-10 minutes. Flip in between.
6. Serve warm with scallions on top.

NUTRITION: Calories: 238; Fat: 13g; Phosphorus: 220mg; Potassium: 348mg; Sodium: 74mg; Carbohydrates: 10g; Protein: 16g.

28. Tuna Casserole

Preparation Time: 15 minutes

Cooking Time: 35 minutes

Serving: 1

INGREDIENTS:

- ½ cup Cheddar cheese, shredded
- 2 tomatoes, chopped
- 7 oz tuna filet, chopped
- 1 teaspoon ground coriander
- ½ teaspoon salt
- 1 teaspoon olive oil
- ½ teaspoon dried oregano

DIRECTIONS:

1. Brush the casserole mold with olive oil.
2. Mix together chopped tuna fillet with dried oregano and ground coriander.
3. Place the fish in the mold and flatten well to get the layer.
4. Then add chopped tomatoes and shredded cheese.
5. Cover the casserole with foil and secure the edges.

6. Bake the meal for 35 minutes at 3550 F.

NUTRITION: Calories 260; Fat 21.5; Phosphorus: 56mg; Potassium: 64mg; Sodium: 29mg; Fiber 0.8; Carbs 2.7; Protein 14.6.

29. Oregano Salmon with Crunchy Crust

Preparation Time: 10 minutes

Cooking Time: 2 hours

Serving: 2

INGREDIENTS:

- 8 oz salmon fillet
- 2 tablespoons panko breadcrumbs
- 1 oz Parmesan, grated
- 1 teaspoon dried oregano
- 1 teaspoon sunflower oil

DIRECTIONS:

1. In the mixing bowl combine panko breadcrumbs, Parmesan, and dried oregano.
2. Sprinkle the salmon with olive oil and coat in the breadcrumb's mixture.
3. After this, line the baking tray with baking paper.
4. Place the salmon in the tray and transfer to the oven preheated at 3850 F.
5. Bake the salmon for 25 minutes.

NUTRITION: Calories 245Kcal; Fat 12.8g; Phosphorus: 30mg; Potassium: 67mg; Sodium: 31mg; Fiber 0.6g; Carbs 5.9g; Protein 27.5g.

30. Sardine Fish Cakes

Preparation Time: 10 minutes

Cooking Time: 10 minutes

Serving: 1

INGREDIENTS:

- 11 oz sardines, canned, drained
- 1/3 cup shallot, chopped
- 1 teaspoon chili flakes
- ½ teaspoon salt

- 2 tablespoon wheat flour, whole grain
- 1 egg, beaten
- 1 tablespoon chives, chopped
- 1 teaspoon olive oil
- 1 teaspoon butter

DIRECTIONS:
1. Put the butter in the skillet and melt it.
2. Add shallot and cook it until translucent.
3. After this, transfer the shallot in the mixing bowl.
4. Add sardines, chili flakes, salt, flour, egg, chives, and mix up until smooth with the help of the fork.
5. Make the medium size cakes and place them in the skillet.
6. Add olive oil.
7. Roast the fish cakes for 3 minutes from each side over the medium heat.
8. Dry the cooked fish cakes with the paper towel if needed and transfer in the serving plates.

NUTRITION: Calories 221; Fat 12.2; Phosphorus: 36mg; Potassium: 194mg; Sodium: 31mg; Fiber 0.1; Carbs 5.4; Protein 21.3

31. Cajun Catfish

Preparation Time: 10 minutes

Cooking Time: 10 minutes

Serving: 1

INGREDIENTS:
- 16 oz catfish steaks (4 oz each fish steak)
- 1 tablespoon Cajun spices
- 1 egg, beaten
- 1 tablespoon sunflower oil

DIRECTIONS:
1. Heat oil in a pan.
2. Meanwhile, dip every catfish steak in the beaten egg and coat in Cajun spices.
3. Place the fish steaks in the hot oil and roast them for 4 minutes from each side.
4. The cooked catfish steaks should have a light brown crust.

NUTRITION: Calories 263; Fat 16.7; Phosphorus: 39mg; Potassium: 74mg; Sodium: 20mg; Fiber 0; Carbs 0.1;

Protein 26.3.

32. Poached Gennaro/Sea Bass with Red Peppers

Preparation Time: 10 minutes

Cooking Time: 40 minutes

Serving: 1

INGREDIENTS:

- 2 red peppers, trimmed
- 11 oz Gennaro/Sea bass, trimmed
- 1 teaspoon salt
- ½ teaspoon ground black pepper
- 2 tablespoons butter
- 1 lemon

DIRECTIONS:

1. Remove the seeds from red peppers and cut them into wedges.
2. Then line the baking tray with parchment and arrange red peppers in a layer.
3. Rub Gennaro/Sea bass with ground black pepper and salt and place it on the peppers.
4. Then add butter.
5. Cut the lemon on the halves and squeeze the juice over the fish.
6. Bake the fish for 40 minutes at 3500 F.

NUTRITION: Calories 148, Fat 10.3, Phosphorus: 36mg; Potassium: 194mg; Sodium: 31mg; Fiber 1.2, Carbs 7.3, Protein 8.5.

33. Shrimp Skewers with Mango Cucumber Salsa

Preparation Time: 10 minutes plus 30 minutes to marinate

Cooking Time: 15 minutes

Serving: 6

INGREDIENTS:

FOR THE SHRIMP

- Juice of 2 limes
- 2 tablespoons honey

- 1-inch piece ginger, minced
- 1 pound large shrimp, peeled and deveined, tails intact
- 1 teaspoon canola oil

FOR THE SALSA

- ¼ cup diced sweet onion
- 1 small red chile, finely diced
- 1 medium cucumber, seeded and diced
- 1 mango, peeled and diced
- Juice of 1 lime

DIRECTIONS:

TO MAKE THE SHRIMP

1. In a medium bowl, combine the lime juice, honey, and ginger. Add the shrimp and toss to coat.
2. Cover and refrigerate for 30 minutes to marinate.
3. Thread the shrimp on skewers.
4. Heat a grill or grill pan over medium-high heat and brush with oil. Cook the skewers 3 to 6 minutes on each side, until the shrimp are opaque and cooked through.

TO MAKE THE SALSA

1. In a small bowl, toss the onion, chile, cucumber, mango, and lime juice.
2. Add the shrimp and toss to coat.
3. Cooking tip: If you don't have a grill pan, you can cook the skewers for 10 to 12 minutes on a rimmed baking dish in a preheated 425°F oven.

NUTRITION: Calories: 123; Total Fat: 2g; Saturated Fat: 0g; Cholesterol: 95mg; Carbohydrates: 17g; Fiber: 3g; Protein: 11g; Phosphorus: 213mg; Potassium: 317mg; Sodium: 431mg

POULTRY

34. Roasted Citrus Chicken

Preparation Time: 20 Minutes

Cooking Time: 60 Minutes

Servings: 8

INGREDIENTS:

- 1 tablespoon olive oil
- 2 cloves garlic, minced
- 1 teaspoon Italian seasoning
- ½ teaspoon black pepper
- 8 chicken thighs
- 2 cups chicken broth, reduced sodium
- 3 tablespoons lemon juice
- ½ large chicken breast for 1 chicken thigh

DIRECTIONS:

1. Warm oil in a huge skillet.
2. Include garlic and seasonings.
3. Include chicken bosoms and dark-colored all sides.
4. Spot chicken in the moderate cooker and include the chicken soup.
5. Cook on LOW heat for 6 to 8 hours.
6. Include lemon juice toward the part of the bargain time.

NUTRITION: Calories 265, Fat 19g, Protein 21g, Carbohydrates 1g

35. Chicken with Asian Vegetables

Preparation Time: 10 Minutes

Cooking Time: 20 Minutes

Servings: 8

INGREDIENTS:

- 2 tablespoons canola oil
- 6 boneless chicken breasts
- 1 cup low-sodium chicken broth

- 3 tablespoons reduced-sodium soy sauce
- ¼ teaspoon crushed red pepper flakes
- 1 garlic clove, crushed
- 1 can (8ounces) water chestnuts, sliced and rinsed (optional)
- ½ cup sliced green onions
- 1 cup chopped red or green bell pepper
- 1 cup chopped celery
- ¼ cup cornstarch
- ⅓ cup water
- 3 cups cooked white rice
- ½ large chicken breast for 1 chicken thigh

DIRECTIONS:

1. Warm oil in a skillet and dark-colored chicken on all sides.
2. Add chicken to a slow cooker with the remainder of the fixings aside from cornstarch and water.
3. Spread and cook on LOW for 6 to 8hours
4. Following 6-8 hours, independently blend cornstarch and cold water until smooth. Gradually include into the moderate cooker.
5. At that point turn on high for about 15mins until thickened. Don't close the top on the moderate cooker to enable steam to leave.
6. Serve Asian blend over rice.

NUTRITION: Calories 415, Fat 20g, Protein 20g, Carbohydrates 36g

36. Chicken Adobo

Preparation Time: 10 Minutes

Cooking Time: 40 Minutes

Servings: 6

INGREDIENTS:

- 4 medium yellow onions, halved and thinly sliced
- 4 medium garlic cloves, smashed and peeled
- 1 (5-inch) piece fresh ginger, cut into1-inch pieces
- 1 bay leaf
- 3 pounds bone-in chicken thighs

- 3 tablespoons reduced-sodium soy sauce
- ¼ cup rice vinegar (not seasoned)
- 1 tablespoon granulated sugar
- ½ teaspoon freshly ground black pepper

DIRECTIONS:
1. Spot the onions, garlic, ginger, and bay leaf in an even layer in the slight cooker.
2. Take out and do away with the pores and skin from the chicken.
3. Organize the hen in an even layer over the onion mixture.
4. Whisk the soy sauce, vinegar, sugar, and pepper collectively in a medium bowl and pour it over the fowl.
5. Spread and prepare dinner on LOW for 8 hours
6. Remove and take away the ginger portions and inlet leaves.
7. Serve with steamed rice.

NUTRITION: Calories 318, Fat 9g, Protein 14g, Carbohydrates 44g

37. Chicken and Veggie Soup

Preparation Time: 15 Minutes

Cooking Time: 25 Minutes

Servings: 8

INGREDIENTS:
- 4 cups cooked and chopped chicken
- 7 cups reduced-sodium chicken broth
- 1-pound frozen white corn
- 1 medium onion diced
- 4 cloves garlic minced
- 2 carrots peeled and diced
- 2 celery stalks chopped
- 2 teaspoons oregano
- 2 teaspoon curry powder
- ½ teaspoon black pepper

DIRECTIONS:
1. Include all fixings into the moderate cooker.

2. Cook on LOW for 8 hours
3. Serve over cooked white rice.

NUTRITION: Calories 220, Fat 7g, Protein 24g, Carbohydrates 19g

38. Turkey Sausages

Preparation Time: 10 Minutes

Cooking Time: 10 Minutes

Servings: 2

INGREDIENTS:

- 1/4 teaspoon salt
- 1/8 teaspoon garlic powder
- 1/8 teaspoon onion powder
- 1 teaspoon fennel seed
- 1 pound 7% fat ground turkey

DIRECTIONS:

1. Press the fennel seed and in a small cup put together turkey with fennel seed, garlic, and onion powder, and salt.
2. Cover the bowl and refrigerate overnight.
3. Prepare the turkey with seasoning into different portions with a circle form and press them into patties ready to be cooked.
4. Cook at medium heat until browned.
5. Cook it for 1 to 2 minutes per side and serve them hot. Enjoy!

NUTRITION: Calories 55, Protein 7 g, Sodium 70 mg, Potassium 105 mg, Phosphorus 75 mg

39. Rosemary Chicken

Preparation Time: 10 Minutes

Cooking Time: 10 Minutes

Servings: 2

INGREDIENTS:

- 2 zucchinis
- 1 carrot
- 1 teaspoon dried rosemary

- 4 chicken breasts
- 1/2 bell pepper
- 1/2 red onion
- 8 garlic cloves
- Olive oil
- 1/4 tablespoon ground pepper

DIRECTIONS:

1. Prepare the oven and preheat it at 375°F (or 200°C).
2. Slice both zucchini and carrots and add bell pepper, onion, garlic, and put all the ingredients, adding oil in a 13" x 9" pan.
3. Spread the pepper on the pan and roast for about 10 minutes.
4. Meanwhile, lift the chicken skin and spread black pepper and rosemary on the flesh.
5. Remove the vegetable pan from the oven and add the chicken, returning the pan to the oven for about 30 more minutes. Serve and enjoy!

NUTRITION: Calories 215, Protein 28 g, Sodium 105 mg, Potassium 580 mg, Phosphorus 250 mg

40. Smokey Turkey Chili

Preparation Time: 5 Minutes

Cooking Time: 45 Minutes

Servings: 8

INGREDIENTS:

- 12-ounce lean ground turkey
- 1/2 red onion, chopped
- 2 cloves garlic, crushed and chopped
- ½ teaspoon of smoked paprika
- ½ teaspoon of chili powder
- ½ teaspoon of dried thyme
- ¼ cup reduced-sodium beef stock
- ½ cup of water
- 1½ cups baby spinach leaves, washed
- 3 wheat tortillas

DIRECTIONS:

1. Brown the ground beef in a dry skillet over medium-high heat.
2. Add in the red onion and garlic.
3. Sauté the onion until it goes clear.
4. Transfer the contents of the skillet to the slow cooker.
5. Add the remaining ingredients and simmer on low for 30–45 minutes.
6. Stir through the spinach for the last few minutes to wilt.
7. Slice tortillas and gently toast under the broiler until slightly crispy.
8. Serve on top of the turkey chili.

NUTRITION: Calories 93.5, Protein 8g, Carbohydrates 3g, Fat 5.5g, Cholesterol 30.5mg, Sodium 84.5mg, Potassium 142.5mg, Phosphorus 92.5mg, Calcium 29mg, Fiber 0.5g

41. Chicken Kebab Sandwich

Preparation Time: 15 Minutes

Cooking Time: 15 Minutes

Servings: 4

INGREDIENTS:

- 12 ounces boneless, skinless chicken breast
- 2 tablespoons freshly squeezed lemon juice
- 1 tablespoon extra-virgin olive oil
- 4 garlic cloves, minced, divided
- Freshly ground black pepper
- ¼ cup plain, unsweetened yogurt
- 4 white flatbreads
- 1 cucumber, sliced
- 1 cup lettuce, shredded

DIRECTIONS:

1. In a medium bowl, add the chicken breast, lemon juice, olive oil, and half the garlic, tossing to coat. Season with pepper. Set aside to marinate while you prepare the other ingredients.
2. In a small bowl, add the yogurt and remaining garlic. Season with pepper and mix well. Set aside.
3. Heat a large skillet over medium-high heat, and add the chicken and the marinade. Cook for 5 minutes, until the chicken is well browned on the underside. Flip it over and cook the other side until the chicken

is golden brown and the juices run clear. Remove from the pan and let rest for 5 minutes. Cut the chicken into thin slices.

4. In each flatbread, add some chicken, cucumber, and lettuce. Top with the yogurt sauce, and serve.
5. Lower sodium tip: Reduce the amount of chicken breast to 8 ounces to lower this dish to 275mg and 15g of protein.

Nutrition Per Serving Calories: 217; Total Fat: 6g; Saturated Fat: 1g; Cholesterol: 49mg; Carbohydrates: 21g; Fiber: 1g; Protein: 22g; Phosphorus: 80mg; Potassium: 231mg; Sodium: 339mg

42. Aromatic Chicken and Cabbage Stir-Fry

Preparation Time: 10 Minutes

Cooking Time: 10 Minutes

Servings: 4

INGREDIENTS:

- 1 teaspoon canola oil
- 10 ounces boneless, skinless chicken breast, thinly sliced
- 3 cups green cabbage, thinly sliced
- 1 tablespoon cornstarch
- 1 teaspoon ground ginger
- ½ teaspoon garlic powder
- ¼ cup water
- Freshly ground black pepper

DIRECTIONS:

1. In a large skillet over medium-high heat, heat the oil. Add the chicken and cook, stirring often, until browned and cooked through.
2. Add the cabbage to the pan, and cook for another 2 to 3 minutes, until the cabbage is tender but still crisp and green.
3. In a small bowl, mix the cornstarch, ginger, garlic, and water. Add the mixture to the pan, and continue cooking until the sauce has slightly thickened, about 1 minute. Season with pepper.
4. Substitution tip: Collards, turnip greens, or mustard greens can be used in this stir-fry in place of cabbage. Because the cooking time is short, remove any tough stems to ensure even cooking.

NUTRITION PER SERVING Calories: 96; Total Fat: 2g; Saturated Fat: 0g; Cholesterol: 38mg; Carbohydrates: 5g; Fiber: 1g; Protein: 15g; Phosphorus: 15mg; Potassium: 140mg; Sodium: 156mg

MEAT

43. Mouthwatering Beef and Chilli Stew

Preparation Time: 15 minutes

Cooking Time: 7 Hours

Servings: 6

INGREDIENTS:

- 1/2 medium red onion, thinly sliced into half moons
- 1/2 tbsp. vegetable oil
- 10oz of flat cut beef brisket, whole
- ½ cup low sodium stock
- ¾ cup water
- ½ tbsp. honey
- ½ tbsp. chili powder
- ½ tsp. smoked paprika
- ½ tsp. dried thyme
- 1 tsp. black pepper
- 1 tbsp. corn starch

DIRECTIONS:

1. Throw the sliced onion into the slow cooker first.
2. Add a splash of oil to a large hot skillet and briefly seal the beef on all sides.
3. Remove the beef from the skillet and place in the slow cooker.
4. Add the stock, water, honey and spices to the same skillet that you cooked the beef in.
5. Loosen the browned bits from the bottom of the pan with spatula. (Hint: These brown bits at the bottom are called the fond.)
6. Allow juice to simmer until the volume is reduced by about half.
7. Pour the juice over beef in the slow cooker.
8. Set the slow cooker on Low and cook for approximately 7 hours.
9. Take the beef out of the slow cooker and onto a platter.
10. Shred it with two forks.
11. Pour the remaining juice into a medium saucepan. Bring to a simmer.
12. Whisk the cornstarch with two tbsp. of water.

13. Add to the juice and cook until slightly thickened.
14. For a thicker sauce, simmer and reduce the juice a bit more before adding cornstarch.
15. Pour the sauce over the meat and serve.

NUTRITION: Calories 128, Protein 13g, Carbohydrates 6g, Fat 6g, Cholesterol 39mg, Sodium 228mg, Potassium 202mg, Phosphorus 119mg, Calcium 16mg, Fiber 1g

44. Beef and Three Pepper Stew

Preparation Time: 15 minutes

Cooking Time: 6 hours

Servings: 6

INGREDIENTS:

- 10oz of flat cut beef brisket, whole
- 1 tsp. of dried thyme
- 1 tsp. of black pepper
- 1 clove garlic
- ½ cup of green onion, thinly sliced
- ½ cup low sodium chicken stock
- 2 cups water
- 1 large green bell pepper, sliced
- 1 large red bell pepper, sliced
- 1 large yellow bell pepper, sliced
- 1 large red onion, sliced

DIRECTIONS:

1. Combine the beef, thyme, pepper, garlic, green onion, stock and water in a slow cooker.
2. Leave it all to cook on High for 4-5 hours until tender.
3. Remove the beef from the slow cooker and let it cool.
4. Shred the beef with two forks and remove any excess fat.
5. Place the shredded beef back into the slow cooker.
6. Add the sliced peppers and the onion.
7. Cook on High for 45 to 60 minutes until the vegetables are tender.

NUTRITION: Calories 132, Protein 14g, Carbohydrates 9g, Fat 5g, Cholesterol 39mg, Sodium 179mg, Potassium 390mg, Phosphorus 141mg, Calcium 33mg, Fiber 2

45. Sticky Pulled Beef Open Sandwiches

Preparation Time: 15 minutes

Cooking Time 5 hours

Servings: 5

INGREDIENTS:

- ½ cup of green onion, sliced
- 2 garlic cloves
- 2 tbsp. of fresh parsley
- 2 large carrots
- 7oz of flat cut beef brisket, whole
- 1 tbsp. of smoked paprika
- 1 tsp. dried parsley
- 1 tsp. of brown sugar
- ½ tsp. of black pepper
- 2 tbsp. of olive oil
- ¼ cup of red wine
- 8 tbsp. of cider vinegar
- 3 cups of water
- 5 slices white bread
- 1 cup of arugula to garnish

DIRECTIONS:

1. Finely chop the green onion, garlic and fresh parsley.
2. Grate the carrot.
3. Put the beef in to roast in a slow cooker.
4. Add the chopped onion, garlic and remaining ingredients, leaving the rolls, fresh parsley and arugula to one side.
5. Stir in the slow cooker to combine.
6. Cover and cook on Low for 8 to 10 hours, or on High for 4 to 5 hours until tender. (Hint: Test for tenderness by pressing into the meat with a fork.)
7. Remove the meat from the slow cooker.
8. Shred it apart with two forks.
9. Return the meat to the broth to keep it warm until ready to serve.

10. Lightly toast the bread and top with shredded beef, arugula, fresh parsley and ½ spoon of the broth.
11. Serve.

NUTRITION: Calories 273, Protein 15g, Carbohydrates 20g, Fat 11g, Cholesterol 37mg, Sodium 308mg, Potassium 399mg, Phosphorus 159mg, Calcium 113mg, Fiber 3g

46. Herby Beef Stroganoff and Fluffy Rice

Preparation Time: 15 minutes

Cooking Time: 5 hours

Servings: 6

INGREDIENTS:

- ½ cup onion
- 2 garlic cloves
- 9oz of flat cut beef brisket, cut into 1" cubes
- ½ cup of reduced-sodium beef stock
- 1/3 cup red wine
- ½ tsp. dried oregano
- ¼ tsp. freshly ground black pepper
- ½ tsp. dried thyme
- ½ tsp. of saffron
- ½ cup almond milk (unenriched)
- ¼ cup all-purpose flour
- 1 cup of water
- 2 ½ cups of white rice

DIRECTIONS:

1. Chop up the onion and mince the garlic cloves.
2. Mix the beef, stock, wine, onion, garlic, oregano, pepper, thyme and saffron in your slow cooker.
3. Cover and cook on High until the beef is tender, for about 4-5 hours.
4. Combine the almond milk, flour and water.
5. Whisk together until smooth.
6. Add the flour mixture to the slow cooker.
7. Cook for another 15 to 25 minutes until the Stroganoff is thick.

8. Cook the rice using the package instructions, leaving out salt.
9. Drain off the excess water.
10. 1Serve the Stroganoff over the rice.

NUTRITION: Calories 241, Protein 15g, Carbohydrates 29g, Fat 5g, Cholesterol 39g, Sodium 182mg, Potassium 206mg, Phosphorus 151mg, Calcium 59mg, Fiber 1g

47. Chunky Beef and Potato Slow Roast

Preparation Time: 15 minutes

Cooking Time: 5-6 hours

Servings: 12

INGREDIENTS:

- 3 cups of peeled potatoes, chunked
- 1 cup of onion
- 2 garlic cloves, chopped
- 1 ¼ pounds flat cut beef brisket, fat trimmed
- 2 of cups water
- 1 tsp. of chili powder
- 1 tbsp. of dried rosemary
- For the sauce:
- 1 tbsp. of freshly grated horseradish
- ½ cup of almond milk (unenriched)
- 1 tbsp. lemon juice (freshly squeezed)
- 1 garlic clove, minced
- A pinch of cayenne pepper

DIRECTIONS:

1. Double boil the potatoes to reduce their potassium content.
2. (Hint: Bring your potato to the boil, then drain and refill with water to boil again.)
3. Chop the onion and the garlic.
4. Place the beef brisket in a slow cooker.
5. Combine water, chopped garlic, chili powder and rosemary
6. Pour the mixture over the brisket.

7. Cover and cook on High for 4-5 hours until the meat is very tender.
8. Drain the potatoes and add them to the slow cooker.
9. Turn heat to High and cook covered until the potatoes are tender.
10. Prepare the horseradish sauce by whisking together horseradish, milk, lemon juice, minced garlic and cayenne pepper.
11. Cover and refrigerate.
12. Serve your casserole with a dash of horseradish sauce on the side.

NUTRITION: Calories 199, Protein 21g, Carbohydrates 12g, Fat 7g, Cholesterol 63mg, Sodium 282mg, Potassium 317, Phosphorus 191mg, Calcium 23mg, Fiber 1g

48. Chinese-style Beef Stew

Preparation Time: 15 minutes

Cooking Time: 6-8 hours

Servings: 6

INGREDIENTS:

- 2 medium carrots
- 2 green onions
- 2 celery stalks
- 1 medium green bell pepper, sliced
- 1 garlic clove
- 8 oz. of canned bean sprouts
- 8 oz. of canned water chestnuts
- 2 tbsp. of coconut oil
- 12oz lean casserole beef, cut into cubes
- ½ cup low-sodium beef stock
- 1 tbsp. brown sugar
- 1/4 cup white wine vinegar
- 1 red chili, finely diced
- 1 ½ cups of water
- 3 cups cooked white rice

DIRECTIONS:

1. Slice the carrots, green onions, celery and green pepper.

2. Crush the garlic. (Hint: Use the flat edge of a knife to do this easily.)
3. Rinse and slice the bamboo shoots and water chestnuts.
4. Heat the coconut oil in a skillet and just brown the beef all over.
5. Transfer the beef to the slow cooker.
6. Add all the ingredients except the water.
7. Stir, then cover and cook on Low for 6 to 8 hours.
8. Turn the slow cooker up to High.
9. Add the cold water to the slow cooker.
10. Stir it in to make it smooth, and leave the cooker lid slightly open.
11. Cook for a further 15 minutes.
12. 1Serve your dish over a bed of rice.

NUTRITION: Calories 267, Protein 14g, Carbohydrates 31g, Fat 9g, Cholesterol 35mg, Sodium 166mg, Potassium 319mg, Phosphorus 148mg, Calcium 41mg, Fiber 3g

49. Beef One-Pot Slow Roast

Preparation Time: 15 minutes

Cooking Time: 4-5 hours

Servings: 8

INGREDIENTS:

- 1 tbsp. plain flour
- 1 pound of boneless beef chuck or rump roast
- 1 tbsp. of olive oil
- ¼ cup leek, sliced
- 2 garlic cloves, minced
- ½ cup rutabaga, peeled and cubed
- ½ tsp. of dried thyme
- 1/2 tsp. of dried parsley
- 1 ½ cups water
- ¼ cup of carrots, sliced

DIRECTIONS:

1. First, dust the beef in flour.

2. In a hot oiled skillet, brown the meat on all sides.
3. Add the onions, then cover and cook on Low for 15 minutes.
4. Add the garlic, rutabaga, herb seasoning and 2 cups of water.
5. Add to the slow cooker and simmer on a medium heat for 3 ½ to 4 hours, until the meat is tender.
6. Finally, add in the carrots and cook for an additional 30 minutes.

NUTRITION: Calories 100, Protein 12g, Carbohydrates 2.5g, Fat 4g, Cholesterol 35.5mg, Sodium 25.5mg, Potassium 149mg, Phosphorus 82.5mg, Calcium 19mg, Fiber 0.5g

50. Pineapple and Mint Lamb Chops

Preparation Time: 15 minutes

Cooking time: 10 minutes

Servings: 4

INGREDIENTS:

- 1/2 tablespoon olive oil
- 2 tablespoons pineapple juice
- ¼ tablespoon chopped fresh mint
- Salt and pepper to taste
- 4 lamb chops

DIRECTIONS:

1. Stir together olive oil, pineapple juice, and mint in a small bowl.
2. Season with salt and pepper to taste.
3. Place lamb chops in a shallow dish, and brush with the olive oil mixture.
4. Marinate in the refrigerator for 1 hour.

NUTRITION: Calories 137, Total Fat 6.4g, Cholesterol 57mg, Sodium 49mg, Total Carbohydrate 0.8g, Total Sugar: 0.7g, Protein 18g, Calcium 9mg, Iron 2mg, Potassium 230mg, Phosphorus 100mg

51. Spiced Lamb Burgers

Preparation Time: 15 minutes

Cooking time: 20 minutes

Servings: 2

INGREDIENTS:

- 1 tbsp. extra virgin olive oil

- 1 tsp. cumin
- ½ finely diced red onion
- 1 minced garlic clove
- 1 tsp. harass spices
- 1 cup arugula
- 1 juiced lemon
- 6 oz. lean ground lamb
- 1 tbsp. parsley
- ½ cup low-fat plain yogurt

DIRECTIONS:
1. Preheat the broiler on a medium to high heat.
2. Mix the ground lamb, red onion, parsley, harass spices, and olive oil until combined. Shape 1-inch thick patties using wet hands.
3. Add the patties to a baking tray and place under the broiler for 7-8 minutes on each side or until thoroughly cooked through.
4. Mix the yogurt, lemon juice, and cumin and serve over the lamb burgers with a side salad of arugula.

NUTRITION: Calories 306, Fat 20g, Carbs 10g, Phosphorus 269mg, Potassium 492mg, Sodium 86mg, Protein 23g

52. Roast Beef

Preparation Time: 15 minutes

Cooking time: 55 minutes

Servings: 3

INGREDIENTS:
- Quality rump or sirloin tip roast

DIRECTIONS:
1. Place in a roasting pan on a shallow rack.
2. Season with pepper and herbs.
3. Insert meat thermometer in the center or thickest part of the roast.
4. Roast to the desired degree of doneness.
5. After removing it from the oven for about 15 minutes, let it chill.
6. In the end, the roast should be moist.

NUTRITION: Calories 158, Protein 24g, Fat 6g, Carbs 0g, Phosphorus 206mg, Potassium 328mg, Sodium 55mg

53. Pork Peccadillo

Preparation Time: 15 minutes

Cooking time: 20 minutes

Servings: 4

INGREDIENTS:

- 2 tablespoons olive oil
- 1 onion, diced, 2 cloves garlic, crushed
- 2 1/2 pounds ground pork
- Salt and pepper to taste
- 1 yellow bell pepper, cut into thin strips
- 1 green bell pepper, cut into thin strips
- 1 red bell pepper, cut into thin strips
- ½ cup kale, chopped

DIRECTIONS:

1. Heat the olive oil in a large skillet over medium heat. Cook and stir the onion and garlic in the oil until tender, about 5 minutes. Remove the onion and garlic from the pan and set aside.
2. Crumble the pork into the skillet and cook until no longer pink. Return the onion and garlic to the skillet and stir through the pork. Season with salt and pepper. Cover the skillet and cook the mixture for 5 minutes.
3. Stir the green bell pepper, red bell pepper, yellow bell pepper into the mixture; cover and cook another 5 minutes. Add the kale to the skillet and stir just before serving.

NUTRITION: Calories 163, Total Fat 9g, Saturated Fat 1.6g, Cholesterol 39mg, Sodium 36mg, Total Carbohydrate 6.2g, Protein 14.9g, Calcium 26mg, Iron 1mg, Potassium 367mg, Phosphorus 241mg

54. Chapter 7: Vegetable

Spring vegetables with tofu from the wok

Preparation Time: 20 minutes

Cooking Time: 30 minutes

Servings: 4

INGREDIENTS:

- 500 g green asparagus
- alternatively: 2 yellow or red peppers
- 1 bunch of spring onions
- 350 g pointed cabbage
- 1 bowl of watercress
- 1 package (100 g) mixed sprouts
- 25 g fresh ginger
- 2 cloves of garlic
- 1 dried chili pepper
- 3-4 tbsp soy sauce
- 3 tbsp lime juice
- 4 tbsp oil
- 300 g tofu
- to turn: wholemeal spelled flour

DIRECTIONS:

1. Wash the asparagus, cut off the woody ends, slice the stalks into pieces about 2 cm wide. Wash, core, and, alternatively, cut the peppers into suitable pieces.

2. Clean, wash, and cut the spring onions into pieces. It cleans and washes pointed cabbage, cutting out the stalk. Cut fine cabbage strips. Clean, dry, spin, and wash. Plug them into bits bite-sized. Peel and chop ginger and garlic. Dried chili crumbles. Combine in a bowl, soy sauce, and lime juice. Add the sesame oil.

3. Heat a wok or deep pan with 2 tablespoons of oil. Cut the tofu into bite-sized pieces and mix with some wholemeal flour. Fry in hot oil until brown. Season with salt and pepper. Use kitchen paper to remove/drain. Drain that oil.

4. Heat the remaining wok oil. Fry asparagus for 1-2 minutes while stirring. Fry onions and cabbage and the remaining vegetables for a minute. Combine marinade, fold pieces of tofu. Season with salt and pepper.

NUTRITION: 383 kcal, 24 g fat, 20 g carbohydrates, 22 g protein, 8 g fibbers, 1.7

55. Asparagus and carrot salad with burrata

Preparation Time: 15 minutes

Cooking Time: 15 minutes

Servings: 2

INGREDIENTS:

- 250 g white asparagus
- 250 g green asparagus
- 2 carrots
- 3 tbsp olive oil
- 1 tbsp sunflower seeds
- 1 tbsp lemon juice
- 150 g cherry tomatoes
- 1 handful arugula
- 1 spring onion
- 2 bullets burrata

DIRECTIONS:

1. Peel the asparagus and the lower ends are cut off. Wash the green asparagus and the woody ends are also cut off. Cut it into pieces with the asparagus. Clean, peel, and cut into sticks with the carrots.
2. In a saucepan, heat the oil and fry the asparagus and carrots over medium heat for five minutes. Add the seeds to the sunflower and roast for 3 minutes. Deglaze with lemon juice and add salt and pepper to season the asparagus and carrot mix. Take it off the stove then and let it cool down.
3. Wash the tomatoes and quarter them at the same time. Rocket wash and dry shake. The spring onions are cleaned, washed, and cut into pieces.
4. Mix the tomatoes, rocket, and spring onions with the asparagus, arrange them on plates and serve each with a scoop of burrata.

NUTRITION: Calories 671 kcal (32%), Protein 34 g (35%), Fat 48 g (41%), Carbohydrates 26 g (17%), added sugar 0 g (0%), fibbers 9.4 g (31%)

56. Quinoa salad Winning

Preparation Time: 30 minutes

Cooking Time: 30 minutes

Servings: 4

INGREDIENTS:

- 200 g quinoa
- 1 mango
- 1 cucumber
- 3 tomatoes
- 1 red pepper
- 150 g lamb's lettuce
- 1 red onion
- 2 stems mint
- 150 g feta (45% fat in dry matter)
- 1 tbsp olive oil
- 1 tbsp apple cider vinegar
- salt
- pepper

DIRECTIONS:

1. Rinse the quinoa with cold water, bring to the boil in a saucepan with twice the amount of water and cook over low heat for about 10 minutes. In the meantime, peel the mango, cut from the stone, and dice the pulp. Clean, wash and cut the cucumber, tomatoes, and peppers. Wash the lamb's lettuce and spin dry. Peel and chop the onion. Wash the mint, shake dry, pluck the leaves and cut into strips. Dice the feta.
2. Drain the quinoa, drain and transfer to a bowl. Add the mango, cucumber, tomatoes, bell pepper, lamb's lettuce, onion, mint, and feta and mix. Season the salad with olive oil, apple cider vinegar, salt, and pepper.

NUTRITION: Calories 409 kcal (19%), Protein 15 g (15%), Fat 16 g (14%), Carbohydrates 50 g (33%), added sugar 0 g (0%), fibbers 8.9 g (30%)

57. Spinach Mango Vegetables

Preparation Time: 20 minutes

Cooking Time: 20 minutes

Servings: 2

INGREDIENTS:

- 750 g young spinach leaves
- 200 g spring onions (2 bunch)

- 800 g ripe mango (2 ripe mangoes)
- 2 tbsp germ oil
- 30 g ginger (1 piece)
- 30 g sunflower seeds (2 tbsp)
- 20 g amaranth pops
- salt
- cayenne pepper

DIRECTIONS:

1. Thoroughly wash the spinach, spin it dry and clean.
2. The spring onions are cleaned and washed and cut into pieces about 2 cm wide.
3. The mangoes peel. Slice the stone pulp and cut it into cubes about 1 cm in size.
4. In a saucepan, heat 1 tablespoon of oil and cook the covered spring onions over medium heat for about 5 minutes. Add the spinach and cook for about 5 minutes, covered.
5. Meanwhile, peel the ginger and finely grate it, collecting the juice.
6. Add the spinach to the mango cubes, ginger and ginger juice, and cover and heat for about 3 minutes over medium heat.
7. Meanwhile, in a coated pan, heat the remaining oil. Roast the seeds of the sunflower for 3-4 minutes over low heat, add the pops of amaranth, and heat briefly.
8. Season the salted spinach and mango vegetables and arrange them on a plate. Sprinkle over the vegetables and season the roasted sunflower seeds and amaranth pops with cayenne pepper.

NUTRITION: Calories 240 kcal (11%), Protein 8 g (8%), Fat 10 g (9%), Carbohydrates 27 g (18%), added sugar 0 g (0%), fibbers 9.5 g (32%)

58. Braised Swiss chard with garlic and balsamic vinegar

Preparation Time: 15 minutes

Cooking Time: 15 minutes

Servings: 2

INGREDIENTS:

- 1 large bunch of Swiss chard
- 1 tbsp. to s. olive oil
- 2 cloves of garlic, minced
- 1/4 tsp. red pepper flakes
- 1 tbsp balsamic vinegar or lemon juice

DIRECTIONS:

1. Clean the leaves and cut their base.
2. Add oil and garlic to a preheated skillet. Add the chilies and leaves, then stir over high heat until the leaves are tender. Add vinegar or lemon juice. Serve with crushed pepper.

NUTRITION: Energy: 88 g, Protein: 1.4 g, Carbohydrates: 5.4 g, Total Fat: 7 g, Sodium: 165 mg, Phosphorus: 42 mg, Potassium: 314 mg

59. Snow peas all with thyme

Preparation Time: 15 minutes

Cooking Time: 30 minutes

Servings: 4

INGREDIENTS:

- 2 tbsp. at t. (10 mL) margarine
- 2 tbsp. at t. (10 mL) fresh lemon juice
- Zest of one lemon
- 1 tsp. at t. (5 mL) dried thyme
- ½ pound (250 g) snow peas, trimmed

DIRECTIONS:

1. Melt the margarine in a shallow pot.
2. Combine lemon zest and juice, and thyme set aside.
3. Steam the snow peas for 3 minutes over boiling water or in the microwave on high for 3 minutes until tender.
4. Drain and fold into the mixture.

NUTRITION: 45 g, Proteins: 2 g, Carbohydrates: 5 g, fibbers: 1.7 g, Total Fat: 2.4 g, Sodium: 30 mg, Phosphorus: 42.6 mg, Potassium: 296 mg

60. Cauliflower and fresh dill

Preparation Time: 15 minutes

Cooking Time: 15 minutes

Servings: 2

INGREDIENTS:

- 1 medium cauliflower head

- 2 tbsp. to s. (25 mL) lemon juice
- 1 tbsp. to s. (15 mL) olive oil
- 1/3 cup (75 mL) fresh dill, chopped
- Pepper to taste

DIRECTIONS:
1. The leaves and stems are removed from the cauliflower; the florets are cut.
2. Cook in a large pot of boiling water, cover for 10 minutes or until tender; drain out the cauliflower.
3. Transfer to a dish for serving.
4. Mix the oil with the lemon juice; pour the cauliflower over it and mix.
5. Sprinkle with dill and sprinkle with pepper to taste.

NUTRITION: Energy: 45 g, Proteins: 2 g, Carbohydrates: 5 g, fibbers: 1.7 g, Total Fat: 2.4 g, Sodium: 30 mg, Phosphorus: 42.6 mg, Potassium: 296 mg

61. Cauliflower and Potato Curry

Preparation Time: 10 minutes

Cooking Time: 15 minutes

Servings: 4

INGREDIENTS:
- 2 tablespoons canola oil
- ½ sweet onion, chopped
- 2-inch piece ginger
- 3 garlic cloves, minced
- 1 teaspoon ground turmeric
- 1 teaspoon ground cumin
- 1 small head cauliflower, cut into florets
- 1 medium potato, diced
- 2 small tomatoes, diced
- 1 small green chile, stemmed, seeded, and diced
- ½ cup water
- Juice of ½ lemon
- ¼ cup chopped cilantro leaves

- 1 teaspoon garam masala
- Rice or bread, for serving

DIRECTIONS:

1. In a large pot over medium heat, heat the olive oil. Add the onion and cook, stirring, until softened.
2. Add the ginger and garlic, and cook until fragrant. Stir in the turmeric and cumin. Add the cauliflower, potato, tomatoes, chile, and water. Bring to a simmer, reduce the heat, and cover. Cook, stirring occasionally, for 25 minutes, until the potatoes and cauliflower are tender.
3. Stir in the lemon juice, cilantro, and garam masala. Serve over rice or with bread.
4. Ingredient tip: Garam masala is a spice blend made up of cumin, coriander, cardamom, black pepper, cinnamon, cloves, nutmeg, and other spices—there are countless variations of the mix. Garam masala is typically added with other spices to curries and South Asian dishes to enhance flavor. Because salt is not added to the blend, a store-bought version is fine, or you can mix your own.

NUTRITION PER SERVING Calories: 146; Total Fat: 7g; Saturated Fat: 1g; Cholesterol: 0mg; Carbohydrates: 19g; Fiber: 3g; Protein: 3g; Phosphorus: 65mg; Potassium: 546mg; Sodium: 20mg

62. Tofu Stir Fry

Preparation time: 15 minutes

Cooking time: 20 minutes

Servings: 4

INGREDIENTS:

- 1 teaspoon sugar
- 1 tablespoon lime juice
- 1 tablespoon low sodium soy sauce
- 2 tablespoons cornstarch
- 2 egg whites, beaten
- 1/2 cup unseasoned bread crumbs
- 1 tablespoon vegetable oil
- 16 ounces tofu, cubed
- 1 clove garlic, minced
- 1 tablespoon sesame oil
- 1 red bell pepper, sliced into strips
- 1 cup broccoli florets
- 1 teaspoon herb seasoning blend

- Dash black pepper
- Sesame seeds
- Steamed white rice

DIRECTIONS:

1. Dissolve sugar in a mixture of lime juice and soy sauce. Set aside. In the first bowl, put the cornstarch. Add the egg whites to the second bowl. Place the breadcrumbs in the third bowl. Dip each tofu cubes in the first, second, and third bowls. Pour vegetable oil into a pan over medium heat. Cook tofu cubes until golden.
2. Drain the tofu and set aside.
3. Remove the oil from the pan and add sesame oil. Add garlic, bell pepper, and broccoli.
4. Cook until crisp-tender. Season with the seasoning blend and pepper. Put the tofu back and toss to mix. Pour soy sauce mixture on top and transfer to serving bowls. Garnish with the sesame seeds and serve on top of white rice.

NUTRITION: Calories: 401, Protein: 19g, Sodium: 584mg, Potassium: 317mg, Phosphorus: 177mg, Calcium: 253mg

63. Broccoli Pancake

Preparation time: 10 minutes

Cooking time: 5 minutes

Servings: 4

INGREDIENTS:

- 3 cups broccoli florets, diced
- 2 eggs, beaten
- 2 tablespoons all-purpose flour
- 1/2 cup onion, chopped
- 2 tablespoons olive oil

DIRECTIONS:

1. Boil broccoli in water for 5 minutes. Drain and set aside.
2. Mix egg and flour.
3. Add onion and broccoli to the mixture.
4. Cook the broccoli pancake until brown on both sides.

NUTRITION: Calories: 140, Protein: 6 g, Sodium: 58mg, Potassium: 276mg, Phosphorus: 101mg

64. Carrot Casserole

Preparation time: 10 minutes

Cooking time: 20 minutes

Serving: 8

INGREDIENTS:

- 1 pound carrots, sliced into rounds
- 12 low-sodium crackers
- 2 tablespoons butter
- 2 tablespoons onion, chopped
- 1/4 cup cheddar cheese, shredded

DIRECTIONS:

1. Preheat your oven to 350 degrees F.
2. Boil carrots in a pot of water until tender.
3. Drain the carrots and reserve ¼ cup liquid.
4. Mash carrots.
5. Add all the ingredients into the carrots except cheese.
6. Place the mashed carrots in a casserole dish.
7. Sprinkle cheese on top and bake in the oven for 15 minutes.

NUTRITION: Calories: 97, Protein: 2g, Sodium: 174mg, Potassium: 153mg.

65. Eggplant Fries

Preparation time: 10 minutes

Cooking time: 5 minutes

Servings: 6

INGREDIENTS:

- 2 eggs, beaten
- 1 cup almond milk
- 1 teaspoon hot sauce
- 3/4 cup cornstarch
- 3 teaspoons dry ranch seasoning mix
- 3/4 cup dry bread crumbs

- 1 eggplant, sliced into strips
- 1/2 cup oil

DIRECTIONS:

1. In a bowl, mix eggs, milk, and hot sauce.
2. In a dish, mix cornstarch, seasoning, and breadcrumbs.
3. Dip first the eggplant strips in the egg mixture.
4. Coat each strip with the cornstarch mixture.
5. Pour oil into a pan over medium heat.
6. Once hot, add the fries and cook for 3 minutes or until golden.

NUTRITION: Calories: 234, Protein: 7g, Sodium: 212mg, Potassium: 215mg, Phosphorus: 86mg, Calcium: 70mg

SOUPS AND STEWS

66. Paprika Pork Soup

Preparation time: 5 minutes

Cooking time: 35 minutes

Servings: 2

INGREDIENTS:

- 4 oz. sliced pork loin
- 1 tsp. black pepper
- 2 minced garlic cloves
- 1 cup baby spinach
- 3 cups water
- 1 tbsp. extra-virgin olive oil
- 1 chopped onion
- 1 tbsp. paprika

DIRECTIONS:

1. In a large pot, add the oil, chopped onion and minced garlic.
2. Sauté for 5 minutes on low heat.
3. Add the pork slices to the onions and cook for 7-8 minutes or until browned.
4. Stir in the spinach, reduce heat and simmer for a further 20 minutes or until pork is thoroughly cooked through.
5. Season with pepper to serve.

NUTRITION: Calories 165, Protein 13 g, Carbs 10 g, Fat 9 g, Sodium (Na) 269 mg, Potassium (K) 486 mg, Phosphorus 158 mg

67. Mediterranean Vegetable Soup

Preparation time: 5 minutes

Cooking time: 30 minutes

Servings: 4

INGREDIENTS:

- 1 tbsp. oregano
- 2 minced garlic cloves

- 1 tsp. black pepper
- 1 diced zucchini
- 1 cup diced eggplant
- 4 cups water
- 1 diced red pepper
- 1 tbsp. extra-virgin olive oil
- 1 diced red onion

DIRECTIONS:

1. Soak the vegetables in warm water prior to use.
2. In a large pot, add the oil, chopped onion and minced garlic.
3. Simmer for 5 minutes on low heat.
4. Add the other vegetables to the onions and cook for 7-8 minutes.
5. Add the stock to the pan and bring to a boil on high heat.
6. Stir in the herbs, reduce the heat, and simmer for a further 20 minutes or until thoroughly cooked through.
7. Season with pepper to serve.

NUTRITION: Calories 152, Protein 1g, Carbs 6g, Fat 3g, Sodium (Na) 3mg, Potassium (K) 229mg, Phosphorus 45mg

68. Tofu Soup

Preparation time: 5 minutes

Cooking Time: 10 minutes

Servings: 2

INGREDIENTS:

- 1 tbsp. Miso paste
- 1/8 cup cubed soft tofu
- 1 chopped green onion
- ¼ cup sliced Shiitake mushrooms
- 3 cups Renali stock
- 1 tbsp. soy sauce

DIRECTIONS:

1. In a saucepan, boil the stock on high heat. Reduce heat to medium and let it simmer. Add mushrooms

and cook for another 3 minutes.

2. Mix Soy sauce (reduced salt) and Miso paste in a bowl. Add this mixture and the tofu to the stock. Simmer for nearly 5 minutes and serve with chopped green onion.

NUTRITION: Calories 129, Fat 7.8g, Sodium (Na) 484mg, Potassium (K) 435mg, Protein 11g, Carbs 5.5g, Phosphorus 73.2mg

69. Beef Stew

Preparation time: 10 minutes

Cooking time: 1 hour

Servings: 4

INGREDIENTS:

- 1 pound of Beef Short Rib
- 2 cups of beef broth
- 4 cloves minced garlic
- 100g onion
- 100g carrot
- 100g radishes
- ¼ tsp of Pink Himalayan Salt
- ¼ tsp of pepper
- ½ tsp of xanthan Gum
- 1 tbsp of Butter
- 1 tbsp of coconut oil

DIRECTIONS:

1. On medium-high heat, heat a large saucepan and add coconut oil. Then add short ribs and brown on all sides. Remove from the saucepan and set aside.
2. Chop onions, carrots and radishes into bite sized pieces and mince garlic. Add onions, garlic and butter and cook for a couple of minutes. Once the onions are soft, add the broth and combine. Add the xanthan gum and mix.
3. Allow broth mixture to come to a boil and then transfer the meat back in and cook covered for 30 minutes. Stir frequently scraping the bottom as you stir.
4. After 30 minutes, add the carrots and radishes and cook for 30 more minutes, stirring frequently until it thickens. If you feel the need you can add more broth or some water. Serve warm and enjoy!

NUTRITION: Calories 432.25kcal, Carbohydrates 5.5g, Protein 19.25g, Fat 36.5g, Fiber 1.5g

70. Lamb Stew

Preparation Time: 30 minutes

Cooking Time: 1 hour and 40 minutes

Servings: 6

INGREDIENTS:

- 1 lb. boneless lamb shoulder, trimmed and cubes
- Black pepper to taste
- 1/4 cup all-purpose flour
- 1 tablespoon olive oil
- 1 onion, chopped
- 3 garlic cloves, chopped
- 1/2 cup tomato sauce
- 2 cups low-sodium beef broth
- 1 teaspoon dried thyme
- 2 parsnips, sliced
- 2 carrots, sliced
- 1 cup frozen peas

DIRECTIONS:

1. Season the lamb with pepper
2. Coat it evenly with flour.
3. Pour oil in a pot over medium heat.
4. Cook the lamb and then set aside.
5. Add onion to the pot.
6. Cook for 2 minutes.
7. Add garlic and sauté for 30 seconds.
8. Pour in the broth to deglaze the pot.
9. Add the tomato sauce and thyme.
10. 1Put the lamb back to the pot.
11. 1Bring to a boil and then simmer for 1 hour.
12. 1Add parsnips and carrots.
13. 1Cook for 30 minutes.

14. 1Add green peas and cook for 5 minutes.

NUTRITION: Calories: 156; Total Fat: 11g; Cholesterol: 26mg; Carbohydrates: 17g; Fiber: 3g, Protein: 7g, Phosphorus: 115mg, Potassium: 567mg, Sodium: 148mg

SNACKS

71. Baked Jicama Fries

Preparation Time: 20 minutes

Cooking Time: 30 minutes

Servings: 4

INGREDIENTS:

- 1 pound jicama root
- 2 tablespoons butter
- 1 tablespoon extra-virgin olive oil
- 1 teaspoon chili powder
- 1 teaspoon paprika
- ¼ teaspoon salt
- ⅛ teaspoon freshly ground black pepper
- 2 tablespoons grated Parmesan cheese

DIRECTIONS:

1. Peel the jicama and cut into ½-inch slices. Cut the slices into strips, each about 4 inches long.
2. In a large saucepan, place the jicama strips and cover with water. Bring to a boil, then boil for 9 minutes. Drain the jicama well and transfer to a rimmed baking sheet. Pat the strips with a paper towel until they are dry, so the strips will crisp in the oven.
3. Preheat the oven to 400°F.
4. In a small saucepan, melt the butter with the olive oil. Drizzle over the jicama on the baking sheet. Sprinkle with the chili powder, paprika, salt, and pepper and toss to coat. Spread the strips into a single layer.
5. Bake the jicama fries for 40 to 45 minutes or until they are browned and crisp, turning once with a spatula halfway through the cooking time.
6. Sprinkle with the Parmesan cheese and serve.
7. Make It Easier Tip: You can buy pre cut jicama at many stores. Make sure that you read the ingredients to confirm the package only contains jicama, not any preservatives or seasonings.

NUTRITION: Calories: 140; Total fat: 10g; Saturated fat: 5g; Sodium: 273mg; Phosphorus: 45mg; Potassium: 204mg; Carbohydrates: 11g; Fiber: 6g; Protein: 2g; Sugar: 2g

72. Double-Boiled Sweet Potatoes

Preparation Time: 20 minutes

Cooking Time: 25 minutes

Servings: 4

INGREDIENTS:

- 2 large sweet potatoes, peeled and cut into 1-inch cubes
- 2 tablespoons extra-virgin olive oil
- 2 tablespoons butter
- 1 red onion, chopped
- ¼ cup half-and-half
- 1 tablespoon honey
- ¼ teaspoon salt
- ⅛ teaspoon freshly ground black pepper

DIRECTIONS:

1. In a large saucepan, fill the pot with water to about an inch above the potatoes. Add the sweet potato cubes and bring to a boil. Boil for 10 minutes.
2. Drain the sweet potatoes, discarding the water.
3. In the same saucepan, fill the pot to the same level again. Add the sweet potato cubes and bring to a boil. Boil for 10 to 15 minutes, or until the potatoes are tender.
4. Meanwhile, in a large skillet, heat the olive oil and butter. Add the red onion and cook for 3 to 5 minutes, stirring, until the onion is very tender.
5. Drain the sweet potatoes once more, discarding the water again. Add the sweet potatoes to the skillet along with the half-and-half, honey, salt, and pepper.
6. Mash the potatoes, using an immersion blender or a potato masher, until the desired consistency. Serve.
7. Make It Easier Tip: You can often find cubed sweet potatoes in the produce aisle at the supermarket. All you have to do is cut the cubes into smaller pieces, then proceed with the recipe.

NUTRITION: Calories: 246; Total fat: 14g; Saturated fat: 6g; Sodium: 235mg; Phosphorus: 62mg; Potassium: 201mg; Carbohydrates: 29g; Fiber: 3g; Protein: 2g; Sugar: 13g

73. Fried Shrimps with Sauce

Preparation time: 20 minutes

Cooking time: 15 minutes

Servings: 7 servings and ½ cup of sauce

INGREDIENTS:

- For Shrimps:
- ¾ cup unbleached flour, divided (½ cup + ¼ cup)
- ¾ teaspoon baking powder
- 1 small egg
- 5 ounces' ice-water
- ¼ cup breadcrumbs
- 30g coconut, unsweetened, shredded
- 300g shrimp (14 pcs), peeled with tails on
- ¼ teaspoon black pepper
- ½ cup olive oil
- For Cilantro sauce:
- 1 clove of garlic
- 1 cup cilantro, chopped
- ¼ cup olive oil
- 2 tablespoons lemon, juiced
- ¼ teaspoon black pepper
- 2 tablespoons yogurt
- 1 teaspoon honey

DIRECTIONS:

1. For Cilantro sauce:
2. Blend all the sauce ingredients until smooth.
3. Add water, one teaspoon at a time, until you achieve desired sauce consistency.
4. For Shrimps:
5. In a mixing bowl add ½ cup of the flour and baking powder. Add the egg in the center of the mix.
6. Beat in the ice-water and combine to obtain a smooth batter. Set aside.
7. In a small separate bowl place the remaining ¼ cup flour.
8. Incorporate breadcrumbs and shredded coconut in a third bowl. Stir well and place next to the other two
9. bowls.
10. Season the shrimp with pepper. Coat the shrimp in flour and then dip it into the batter.

11. Roll each shrimp in the breadcrumb mix. Proceed in the same way until all shrimp are coated.
12. Heat the oil on a deep saucepan and fry the shrimps for 2 minutes until golden and crisp. Flip and cook on
13. top side for 1 minute more.
14. Drain onto paper towels Serve the shrimps with cilantro sauce.
15. Serve and enjoy!

NUTRITION: Calories 375, Fat 28 g, Cholesterol 105 mg, Carbohydrates 16 g, Sugar 2 g, Fiber 3 g, Protein 14 g, Sodium 131 mg, Calcium 82 mg, Phosphorus 153 mg, Potassium 186 mg

74. Hard-Boiled Eggs with Onions

Preparation time: 5 minutes

Cooking time: 12 minutes

Serving size: 1 deviled egg

INGREDIENTS:

- For Eggs:
- 6 large eggs, hard-boiled
- 2 tablespoons 2% plain Greek yogurt
- 2 tablespoons avocado mayonnaise
- 1 teaspoon Dijon mustard
- 2 tablespoons pickled red onion, chopped
- For Pickled Onions: - makes 1 cup -
- 1 small red onion, sliced
- ½ cup water
- ½ cup apple cider vinegar
- 1 teaspoon sugar

DIRECTIONS:

1. For Red Onions:
2. Place all the ingredients in a small saucepan and bring to a boil.
3. Reduce to medium heat and softly cook for about 3-5 minutes.
4. Cool and store refrigerated.
5. For Eggs:
6. Peel and slice the hard-boiled eggs in half lengthwise.

7. In a mixing bowl mash the yolks. Add the yogurt, mayonnaise and mustard. Stir well.
8. Fill in the egg whites with the mix prepared.
9. Decorate with the red onions and refrigerate.
10. Serve and enjoy!

NUTRITION: Calories 59, Fat 6 g, Cholesterol 98 mg, Carbohydrate 2 g, Sugar 0 g, Fiber 0 g, Protein 4 g, Sodium 62 mg, Calcium 17 mg, Phosphorus 46 mg, Potassium 39 mg

75. Simple Cookies

Preparation time: 15 minutes + 1h 30 refrigerator

Cooking time: 15 minutes

Servings: 52 cookies

INGREDIENTS:

- 1 cup butter, softened
- 3 ounces cream cheese, softened
- 1 cup sugar
- 1 egg yolk
- 1 teaspoon vanilla extract
- 2½ cups all-purpose white flour
- 16 ounces candied cherry halves

DIRECTIONS:

1. Preheat the oven to 350°F.
2. Blend the butter, cream cheese, and sugar for about 3 minutes until fluffy.
3. Whisk vanilla with egg yolk.
4. Add the flour and mix well until crumbly.
5. Chill the mixture for at least 1 hour.
6. Shape dough into 1 tablespoon-sized balls and place on greased cookie sheets.
7. Decorate with a cherry half into each cookie.
8. Bake for about 15 minutes until cookies are browned.
9. Cool for about 30 minutes.
10. 1Serve and enjoy!

NUTRITION: Calories 106, Fat 5 g, Cholesterol 16 mg, Carbohydrates 15 g, Sugar 5 g, Fiber 2 g, Protein 1 g, Sodium 7 mg, Calcium 7 mg, Phosphorus 13 mg, Potassium 28 mg

76. Popcorn with Sauce

Preparation time: 5 minutes

Cooking time: 5 minutes

Servings: 8

INGREDIENTS:

- ¼ cup popcorn kernels
- 2 tablespoons unsalted butter, melted
- 4 teaspoons sriracha sauce

DIRECTIONS:

1. Heat a big nonstick pan with a fitting lid and when hot, add the popcorn kernels.
2. Place the lid and shake the pan every couple of seconds. The kernels should start popping within 2 minutes. Continue to shake the pan until there is at least a 4 seconds interval in between kernel pops.
3. Cool the popcorn in a medium bowl.
4. In a separate bowl blend the butter with sriracha.
5. Stir the sriracha butter with popcorn.
6. Serve and enjoy!

NUTRITION: Calories 58, Fat 4 g, Cholesterol 9 mg, Carbohydrates 8 g, Sugar 2 g, Fiber 1 g, Protein 1 g, Sodium 72 mg, Calcium 3 mg, Phosphorus 27 mg, Potassium 36 mg

77. Edamame Dip

Preparation time: 10 minutes

Cooking time: 5 minutes

Servings: 2 cups

INGREDIENTS:

- 2 cups shelled edamame, about 2 pounds fresh or frozen
- 1 small lemon, juiced
- 2 cloves roasted garlic
- 1 scallion, chopped
- 2 tablespoons Parmesan cheese, grated
- ¼ cup parsley
- ¼ cup extra-virgin olive oil

DIRECTIONS:

1. Bring to a boil into water the edamame for about 5 minutes, until tender.
2. Drain and set aside ½ cup of liquid to cool.
3. Blend the edamame, lemon juice, garlic, scallion, Parmesan and parsley. While blending slowly add the olive
4. oil and process until smooth.
5. If necessary, add a few tablespoons of cooking liquid at a time to achieve wished consistency.
6. Serve chill and enjoy!

NUTRITION: Calories 31, Fat 2 g, Cholesterol 0 mg, Carbohydrate 2 g, Sugar 0 g, Fiber 2 g, Protein 2 g, Sodium 8 mg, Calcium 12 mg, Phosphorus 22 mg, Potassium 50 mg

78. Moo-Less Chocolate Mousse

Preparation Time: 10 minutes

Cooking Time: 5 minutes

Servings: 2

INGREDIENTS:

- 2 ripe avocados
- 1 ripe banana
- 1/4 cup unsweetened cocoa powder
- 2-4 tbsp coconut milk
- 1-4 tbsp maple syrup
- 1/2 tsp pure vanilla extract
- 1 pinch cinnamon
- 1 pinch sea salt

DIRECTIONS:

1. Scoop out the flesh of the avocados and mash by hand.
2. Add all the ingredients in a blender and process until creamy.
3. Serve in 2 bowls. Garnish with toasted hazelnuts.

NUTRITION: Calories: 346, Carbs: 35g, Fat: 26g, Protein: 6g

79. Baked Carrots

Preparation Time: 40 minutes

Cooking Time: 25 minutes

Servings: 3

INGREDIENTS:

- 1 tbsp butter
- 3 cloves garlic
- Zest and juice of 1 orange
- Handful of fresh parsley leaves
- 1 lb. carrots
- ½ cup extra-virgin olive oil
- 1 cup chicken stock
- Salt and pepper to taste

DIRECTIONS:

1. Mince the garlic.
2. Slice the carrots very thinly.
3. Chop the fresh parsley leaves.
4. Mix in a bowl the garlic, orange zest and parsley.
5. Cover a roasting dish with some butter and put the previous mixture on it.
6. Arrange carrot slices on the bottom, add some olive oil on top, sprinkle with salt, pepper, garlic, zest and parsley mixture.
7. Repeat previous step until you go out of carrots.
8. Add orange juice and chicken stock.
9. Cover with a piece of wax paper. Bake for 20-25 minutes until carrots are fork-tender.

NUTRITION: Calories: 109, Fat: 5.8g, Carbs: 14g, Protein: 1.4g

80. Cranberry & Apple Coleslaw

Preparation Time: 15 minutes

Cooking Time: 10 minutes

Servings: 6

INGREDIENTS:

- ½ lb. cabbage
- ½ lb. shredded carrots
- 2 granny smith apples
- 2 cups fresh or dried cranberries
- 1 cup mayonnaise
- ¼ cup apple cider vinegar
- 2 tbsp honey

DIRECTIONS:

1. Shred the cabbage and carrots.
2. Core and chop the apples in small matchsticks.
3. Combine the mayonnaise, apple cider vinegar and honey in a large bowl.
4. Add the cabbage, carrots, apples and cranberries to the bowl and mix everything together.

NUTRITION: Calories: 109, Fat: 5.8g, Carbs: 14g, Protein: 1.4g

81. Apple and Fennel Salad

Preparation Time: 15 minutes

Servings: 6

INGREDIENTS:

- 1 fennel bulb
- 1 granny smith apple
- 2 tbsp lemon juice
- 3 tbsp extra-virgin olive oil
- Fennel top
- 1/3 tsp mustard

DIRECTIONS:

1. Slice the fennel bulb and apples.
2. Mix the mustard and lemon juice in a bowl and add the olive oil, sea salt and black pepper to taste.
3. Combine the apple and fennel slices in a bowl and pour the vinaigrette over. Add salt and pepper again.
4. Serve and garnish with the chopped fennel top

NUTRITION: Calories: 248, Fat: 10g, Carbs: 36g, Protein: 6g

DESSERTS

82. Lemon Squares

Preparation time: 10 minutes

Cooking Time: 35 minutes

Servings: 12

INGREDIENTS:

- 1 cup powdered sugar
- 1 cup all-purpose white flour
- ½ cup unsalted butter
- 1 cup granulated sugar
- ½ tsp baking powder
- 2 eggs, slightly beaten
- 4 tbsps lemon juice
- 1 tbsp unsalted butter, softened
- 1 tbsp lemon rind, grated

DIRECTIONS:

1. Start mixing ¼ cup confectioner's sugar, ½ cup butter, and flour in a bowl.
2. Spread this crust mixture in an 8-inch square pan and press it.
3. Bake this flour crust for 15 minutes at 350°F.
4. Meanwhile, prepare the filling by beating granulated sugar, 2 tablespoons lemon juice, lemon rind, eggs and baking powder in a mixer.
5. Spread this filling in the baked crust and bake again for 20 minutes.
6. Prepare the icing meanwhile by beating 1 tablespoon butter with 2 tablespoons lemon juice and ¾ cup confectioners' sugar.
7. Once the lemon pie is baked, allow it to cool.
8. Drizzle the icing mixture on top of the lemon pie then cut it into 36 squares.
9. Serve.

NUTRITION: Calories 146, Protein 2g, Carbohydrates 22g, Fat 6g, Cholesterol 39mg, Sodium 45mg, Potassium 22mg, Phosphorus 32mg, Calcium 16mg, Fiber 0.2g

83. Homemade apple sauce

Preparation time: 5 minutes

Cooking time: 40 minutes

Servings: 3

INGREDIENTS:

- 6 pounds of apples, peeled, cored and cut into 8 slices
- 1 cup apple juice or apple cider
- 1 lemon (juice)
- ½ tsp brown sugar
- 1 tsp of cinnamon (more or less to taste)

DIRECTIONS:

1. Combine all the ingredients in a large saucepan and cook over medium heat, stirring occasionally for 25 minutes.
2. Mash gently in a food processor or blender (do not overfill; divide into two portions if necessary) until smooth.

NUTRITION: Calories 124kcal, Potassium 182mg, Sodium 3mg, Phosphorus 20mg, Protein 1g

84. Ice cream sandwiches

Preparation time: 5 minutes

Cooking time: 30 minutes

Servings: 3

INGREDIENTS:

- 10 easy graham crackers
- 20 tbsps non dairy whisk, fresh

DIRECTIONS

1. Break the graham crackers in half.
2. Put 2 tablespoons cold whisk into each half
3. Cover with the other half of the cookie.
4. Place on the dish and freeze for several hours.
5. Wrap individual frozen rolls in Saran Wrap.

NUTRITION: Calories 37kcal, Potassium 18mg, Sodium 36mg, Phosphorus 15mg, Protein 1g

85. Creamy Pineapple Dessert

Preparation time: 10 minutes

Cooking Time: 0 minutes

Servings: 2

INGREDIENTS:

- 16 ounces cottage cheese
- 15 ounces canned pineapple
- 8 ounces whipped topping
- ½ tsp green food coloring

DIRECTION:

1. Throw all the dessert ingredients into a suitably sized bowl.
2. Mix them well and refrigerate for 1 hour.
3. Serve.

NUTRITION: Calories 204, Protein 10g, Carbohydrates 23g, Fat 8g, Cholesterol 13mg, Sodium 303mg, Potassium 203mg, Phosphorus 152mg, Calcium 100mg, Fiber 0.6g

86. Blackberry Mountain Pie

Preparation time: 10 minutes

Cooking Time: 45 minutes

Servings: 8

INGREDIENTS:

- 1/3 cup unsalted butter
- 4 cups blackberries
- 13 tbsps sugar
- 1 cup all-purpose white flour
- ½ tsp baking powder
- ¾ cup Rice Drink

DIRECTION:

1. Preheat the oven to 375°F.
2. Grease a 2-quart baking dish with melted butter.
3. Toss blackberries with 1 tablespoon sugar in a small bowl.

4. Whisk the remaining ingredients in a mixer until they form a smooth batter.
5. Spread this pie batter in the prepared baking dish and top it with blackberries.
6. Bake the blackberry pie for 45 minutes in the preheated oven.
7. Slice and serve once chilled.

NUTRITION: Calories 320, Protein 4g, Carbohydrates 49g, Fat 12g, Cholesterol 28mg, Sodium 222mg, Potassium 186mg, Phosphorus 91mg, Calcium 65mg, Fiber 5.6g

87. Baked Apple Pie

Preparation time: 5 minutes

Cooking Time: 1 hour

Servings: 4

INGREDIENTS:

- 2 cups cooking apples, peeled and sliced
- 2 whole cloves
- 1 tsp cinnamon
- 1 cup breadcrumbs
- 1 tbsp coconut oil

DIRECTIONS:

1. Preheat the oven to 190°C/375°F/Gas Mark 5.
2. Boil a pot of water over a high heat and add the apples, cloves and cinnamon.
3. Turn down the heat slightly and allow to cook for 30-35 minutes or until very soft.
4. Drain and add apples to the bottom of an oven dish.
5. Blitz up the breadcrumbs and add coconut oil to combine.
6. Top the apples with this mixture and place in the oven to bake for 20-30 minutes or until golden brown.

NUTRITION: Calories 36, Protein 0 g, Carbohydrates 20 g, Fat 1 g, Sodium 4 mg, Potassium 566 mg, Phosphorus 55 mg

88. Whipped Strawberry Mousse

Preparation time: 4-5 hours

Cooking Time: 0 minutes

Servings: 4

INGREDIENTS:

- 6oz silken extra firm tofu
- 2 Tbsp rice milk
- 1 Cup fresh strawberries

DIRECTIONS:

1. Blend the tofu, strawberries and milk until smooth (you can use water here instead if you wish).
2. Add the mousse into serving cups and cover and refrigerate for 4-5 hours.
3. Enjoy!

NUTRITION: Calories 131, Protein 7 g, Carbohydrates 8 g, Fat 8 g, Sodium 20 mg, Potassium 120 mg, Phosphorus 10 mg

89. Chocolate Chips Fudge

Preparation time: 5 minutes

Cooking Time: 1 hour 30 minutes

Servings: 2

INGREDIENTS

- 1 cup coconut milk, full-fat
- 1 tbsp vanilla extract
- 2½ cups chocolate chips, sugar-free
- 1-2 tbsps liquid stevia or to taste
- ⅛ tbsp salt

DIRECTIONS:

1. Line a baking dish, 8 x 8 inches, with parchment paper. Set aside.
2. Pour coconut milk into your slow cooker then add vanilla, chocolate chips, stevia, and salt. Stir to combine.
3. Cover using a paper towel then place the lid on a jar, slightly, allowing steam to escape.
4. Cook for about 1½ hours on Low. Turn off then stir until smooth.
5. Transfer and spread the mixture on the baking dish and refrigerate for about 1 hour until firm.
6. Cut the fudge into 25 pieces, equal squares, then store in the fridge for up to 2 weeks in a container, airtight.
7. Serve and enjoy.

Nutritional Facts Per Serving Calories:85, Total fat: 9g, Saturated fat: 3g, Total carbs: 1g, Net carbs: 1g, Protein: 0g, Sugar: 1g, Fiber: 0g, Sodium: 123mg, Potassium: 230mg

90. Chocolate Molten Lava Cake

Preparation time: 10 minutes

Cooking time: 3 hours

Servings: 12

INGREDIENTS

- Cooking spray
- 1 ½ cup swerve
- ½ cup flour, gluten-free
- 5 tbsp cocoa powder, unsweetened and divided
- 1 tbsp baking powder
- ½ tbsp salt
- ½ cup butter, melted
- 3 eggs
- 3 egg yolks
- 1 tbsp vanilla extract
- ½ tbsp vanilla liquid stevia
- 4 oz chocolate chips, sugar-free
- 2 cups hot water

DIRECTIONS:

1. Grease your slow cooker with oil.
2. Whisk together 1 ¼ cup swerve, flour, 3 tbsp cocoa powder, baking powder and salt in a mixing bowl.
3. In another bowl mix butter, eggs, egg yolks, vanilla extract, and vanilla liquid stevia.
4. Add the wet ingredients into the dry ingredients and mix until well combined.
5. Pour mixture into the slow cooker and top with chocolate chips.
6. Whisk together the remaining cocoa powder, swerve and hot water. Pour the mixture over the chocolate chips.
7. Cover the slow cooker and cook for 3 hours on low. Let rest to cool before serving.

NUTRITION: Calories 174.6, Total Fat 13g, Saturated Fat 6.4g, Total Carbs 10.5g, Net Carbs 7.9g, Protein 3.9g, Sugar: 0.2g, Fiber: 2.6g, Sodium: 166mg

91. Coconut Almond Cake

Preparation time: 10 minutes

Cooking time: 4 hours

Servings: 8

INGREDIENTS

- 1 cup almond flour
- ½ cup coconut, unsweetened and shredded
- ⅓ cup stevia
- 1 tbsp baking powder
- 1 tbsp apple pie spice
- 2 eggs, lightly whisked
- ¼ cup butter, melted
- ½ cup heavy whipping cream
- 2 cups of water

DIRECTIONS:

1. Mix all dry ingredients in a mixing bowl until well combined.
2. Add the wet ingredients one at a time ensuring you mix thoroughly with each addition.
3. Pour the mixture in a cake pan that can fit your slow cooker and cover with paper foil.
4. Place two cups of water in your slow cooker and place the trivet in place.
5. Lower the cake pan on the trivet then cover the slow cooker. Cook on high for 4 hours.
6. When the time has elapsed, take out the cake pan and place it on a cooling rack. Let cool for 20 minutes.
7. Transfer the cake to a plate then sprinkle with almonds and coconuts.
8. Serve and enjoy.

NUTRITION: Calories 247, Total Fat 23g, Saturated Fat 11g, Total Carbs 5g, Net Carbs 3g, Protein 5g, Sugar: 3g, Fiber: 2g, Sodium: 74mg, Potassium: 108mg

92. Dark Chocolate Cake

Preparation time: 10 minutes

Cooking time: 3 hours

Servings: 10

INGREDIENTS

- Cooking spray
- 1 cup + 2 tbsp almond flour
- ½ cup swerve granular
- 3 tbsp protein powder, unflavored
- ½ cup cocoa powder, sugar-free
- 1 ½ tbsp baking powder
- ¼ tbsp salt
- 3 eggs
- 6 tbsp butter, melted
- ⅔ cup almond milk, unsweetened
- ¾ tbsp vanilla extract
- ⅓ cup chocolate chips, sugar-free

DIRECTIONS:

1. Grease your 6 -quart slow cooker insert well with oil.
2. Whisk together flour, swerve, protein powder, cocoa powder, baking powder and salt in a mixing bowl.
3. Stir in eggs, butter, milk, vanilla extract, and chocolate chips until well combined.
4. Pour the mixture in the greased slow cooker insert and cook on low for 2 ½ hours.
5. When the time has elapsed, turn off the slow cooker and let the cake rest for 30 minutes before slicing.
6. Serve and enjoy.

NUTRITION: Calories 216.2, Total Fat 17g, Saturated Fat 8g, Total Carbs 8.4g, Net Carbs 4.4g, Protein 7.37g, Sugar: 3g, Fiber: 4.1g, Sodium: 347mg, Potassium 141g

93. Sweet Blueberry Lemon Cake

Preparation time: 10 minutes

Cooking Time: 2 hours and 30 minutes; Servings: 10

INGREDIENTS

- For the sauce
- ¼ cup lemon juice
- 1 ½ cup blueberries
- 1 tbsp monk fruit powder

- ¼ cup ghee
- 2 tbsp water
- 1 tbsp almond flour
- For the cake
- 1 ½ tbsp lemon zest
- ½ cup ghee, melted
- ½ cup coconut cream
- ¼ lemon juice
- 4 eggs
- ¼ cup coconut flour
- 2 cups almond flour
- 2 tbsp baking powder
- 3 tbsp monk fruit powder, divided

DIRECTIONS:

1. For the Blueberry Lemon Sauce
2. Combine the lemon juice, blueberries, monk fruit, and ghee in a small saucepan over medium-high heat until well combined. Bring to boil.
3. Whisk together water and almond flour in a bowl until the flour is dissolved. Pour the mixture over the blueberries mixture and stir to mix.
4. Simmer for about 2 to 4 minutes ensuring you stir occasionally until the sauce thickens.
5. For the cake
6. Whisk together lemon zest, ghee, cream, lemon juice, and eggs in a mixing bowl.
7. Sift in coconut flour, almond flour, baking powder, and fruit powder. Stir until well combined.
8. Pour the cake mixture in the slow cooker insert and smooth it out.
9. Add the blueberry sauce over the cake and gently swirl it using a butter knife tip.
10. Cook on high for 2 ½ hours then serve warm. Enjoy.

NUTRITION: Calories 169, Total Fat 25g, Saturated Fat 8g, Total Carbs 31g, Net Carbs 6g, Protein 10g, Sugar: 12g, Fiber: 13g, Sodium: 50mg, Potassium 71mg

94. Lemon Coconut Cream Dessert

Preparation time: 10 minutes

Cooking time: 3 hours

Servings: 4

INGREDIENTS

- 5 eggs
- ¼ cup lemon juice, freshly squeezed
- 1 tbsp lemon zest
- 1 tbsp vanilla extract
- ½ tbsp liquid stevia
- 2 cups coconut cream
- Whipped cream, slightly sweetened

DIRECTIONS:

1. Whisk together egg yolks, lemon juice and zest, vanilla extract and liquid stevia in a mixing bowl.
2. Whisk in coconut cream until well mixed then divide the mixture among 4 ramekins.
3. Place a rack in the slow cooker and place the ramekins on the rack.
4. Add water to the slow cooker until it reaches halfway up the sides of the ramekins.
5. Cover the slow cooker and cook on low for 3 hours.
6. When the time has elapsed remove the ramekins from the slow cooker and let the custard rest to cool.
7. Top with whipped cream, serve and enjoy.

NUTRITION: Calories 310, Total Fat 30g, Saturated Fat 9g, Total Carbs 3g, Net Carbs 3g, Protein 7g, Sugar: 11g, Fiber: 0g, Sodium: 499mg, Potassium 110g

95. Pumpkin Pie Pudding

Preparation time: 10 minutes

Cooking time: 3 hours

Servings: 6

INGREDIENTS

- 2 eggs
- ½ cup heavy whipping cream
- ¾ cup Erythritol

- 15 oz pumpkin puree, canned
- 1 tbsp pumpkin pie spice
- 1 tbsp vanilla extract
- 1 ½ cup water
- ½ cup heavy whipping cream for finishing

DIRECTIONS:

1. Whisk together eggs with all the other ingredients in the order of listing.
2. Grease a 6x3 inch pan and pour the egg mixture into it.
3. Pour 1 ½ cup water in the slow cooker then place a rack. Place the pan with the mixture on the rack and cover the pan with aluminum foil.
4. Cover the slow cooker and cook for three hours on low.
5. When the time has elapsed, remove the lid carefully so as not to allow any water to fall on the pudding.
6. Remove the pudding from the slow cooker and let rest to cool for 8 hours.
7. Serve with heavy whipping cream. Enjoy.

NUTRITION: Calories 188, Total Fat 16g, Saturated Fat 9g, Total Carbs 8g, Net Carbs 6g, Protein 3g, Sugar: 2g, Fiber 2g, Sodium: 104mg, Potassium 390g

96. Sugar-Free Fudge

Preparation time: 5 minutes

Cooking time: 2 hours

Servings: 30

INGREDIENTS

- 2 ½ cups chocolate chips, sugar-free
- ⅓ cup coconut milk
- 1 tbsp vanilla extract, pure
- Dash of salt
- 2 tbsp vanilla liquid stevia

DIRECTIONS:

1. Stir chocolate chips, coconut milk, vanilla extract, salt, and liquid stevia in a 4-quart slow cooker.
2. Cover the slow cooker and cook for 2 hours on low. When the time has elapsed, turn off the slow cooker and let sit for 30 minutes.
3. Stir until smooth. Line the casserole dish with foil and spread the mixture on it.

4. Chill until firm, cut into 30 pieces and serve.

NUTRITION: Calories 57, Total Fat 5g, Saturated Fat 3g, Total Carbs 2g, Net Carbs 2g, Protein 1g, Sugar: 0g, Fiber: 0g, Sodium: 10mg

97. Peppermint Extract Fudge

Preparation time: 5 minutes

Cooking time: 3 hours

Servings: 18

INGREDIENTS

- 2 ½ cup chocolate chips, sugar-free
- ⅓ cup coconut milk, canned
- 2 tbsp liquid peppermint stevia
- 2 tbsp peppermint extract
- Dash of salt

DIRECTIONS:

1. Add all the ingredients into a 4- quart slow cooker.
2. Cover the slow cooker and cook for 2 hours on low.
3. Uncover the slow cooker and continue cooking for 1 hour. Stir for five minutes until well incorporated.
4. Line a baking dish with foil and pour the chocolate mixture.
5. Refrigerate for 2 hours then transfer to a cutting board. Cut into 18 pieces and serve.

NUTRITION: Calories 77.8, Total Fat 4.6g, Saturated Fat 3.1g, Total Carbs 8.1g, Net Carbs 6.1g, Protein 1g, Sugar: 0.1g, Fiber: 2g, Sodium: 1mg

98. Key Lime Cheesecake

Preparation time: 15 minutes

Cooking time: 7 hours

Servings: 6

INGREDIENTS

- Almond crust
- 1 cup almond flour
- 2 oz butter, melted
- 1 tbsp swerve, granulated

- Key Lime filling
- 18 oz cream cheese
- 1/33 cup swerve, granulated
- 1 tbsp vanilla extract
- 2 oz heavy whipping cream
- 4 tbsp key lime juice
- 2 eggs
- 1 ½ cup of water
- Whipped Cream
- 4 heavy whipping cream
- 1 tbsp swerve, granulated

DIRECTIONS:

1. Almond crust
2. Add all the crust ingredients in a mixing bowl and mix until well combined.
3. spread the mixture in a cake pan that perfectly fits your slow cooker. Press the crust mixture to the bottom of the cake pan then refrigerate until you're ready to use it.
4. Key Lime filling
5. Add all filling ingredients in a mixing bowl except 1 egg. Use a hand mixer to mix until well incorporated.
6. Add the second egg and mix until no yellow from the egg can be seen. Pour mixture over the crust and use a spatula to smooth it out.
7. Tightly cover the cake top and bottom with both paper towels and foil.
8. Add 1 ½ cup of water to the slow cooker and place the rack. Lower the cake pan into the slow cooker.
9. Cover the slow cooker and cook on low for 7 hours. When the time has elapsed, transfer the cake to a cooling rack for 1 hour before refrigerating overnight.
10. Whipped Cream
11. Add cream and swerve to a mixing bowl. Use a hand mixer to mix until stiff peaks form and turn into whipped cream. Refrigerate.
12. Top your cheesecake with whipped cream, serve and enjoy.

NUTRITION: Calories 585, Total Fat 57g, Saturated Fat 9g, Total Carbs 7g, Net Carbs 6g, Protein 11g, Sugar: 3g, Fiber: 1g, Sodium: 365mg, Potassium 158mg

99. Sticky Toffee Pudding

Preparation time: 15 minutes

Cooking time: 6 hours 45 minutes

Servings: 8

INGREDIENTS

- Cake
- 2 tbsp Yacon syrup
- ½ tbsp vanilla extract
- ½ cup hot water
- 1 ½ tbsp cups almond flour
- ½ tbsp cocoa powder
- ½ cup baking soda
- ¼ tbsp salt
- 6 tbsp butter, soft
- ¾ tbsp swerve sweetener
- 2 eggs
- Toffee Sauce
- 6 tbsp butter
- ¼ cup swerve brown
- ¼ cup Bocha sweet
- ½ cup whipping cream, heavy
- ½ tbsp vanilla extract

DIRECTIONS:

1. Line a ceramic souffle dish with a circle parchment paper then grease the parchment paper with oil.
2. Whisk together yacon syrup, vanilla extract and hot water in a mixing bowl. Set aside.
3. In a separate bowl, whisk together flour, cocoa, baking soda, and salt.
4. In another large bowl, beat butter and sweetener until lightened and fluffy. Beat in eggs until combined.
5. Beat in the flour mixture and the yacon syrup mixture until smooth into the large bowl.
6. Spread the batter into the souffle dish then use a spatula to smooth the top. Tightly cover the top with aluminum foil.
7. Add 1 ½ cup of water to the slow cooker and place the trivet. Lower the souffle dish on to the trivet.

8. Cover the slow cooker and cook on low for 6 hours. When the time has elapsed let it rest to firm up completely.
9. Flip out the cake on a serving platter and slice.
10. Toffee sauce
11. Combine butter and sweetener in a skillet over medium heat. Stir cook until they melt and later boil.
12. Reduce heat and continue cooking until it is deep yellow in color. Add whipping cream and vanilla extract to the skillet and whisk until smooth.
13. Let the mixture boil for two minutes.
14. Let rest to cool then serve over cake. Enjoy.

NUTRITION: Calories 348.2, Total Fat 33g, Saturated Fat 10g, Total Carbs 6.2g, Net Carbs 3.8g, Protein 6.6g, Sugar: 3g, Fiber: 2.4g, Sodium: 280mg

100. Spiced Candied Nuts

Preparation time: 5 minutes

Cooking Time: 2-4 hours

Servings: 5

INGREDIENTS

- 3 tbsp vanilla extract
- 2 egg whites
- 1 cup almonds, raw
- 1 cup walnuts, raw
- 1 cup pecans, raw
- 1 cup erythritol
- 1 cup swerve
- 10 drops stevia glycerite
- 2 tbsp cinnamon
- ⅛ tbsp nutmeg
- A pinch cayenne pepper
- ¼ tbsp salt
- ⅓ Cup water

DIRECTIONS:

1. Whip vanilla extract and egg whites in a medium bowl using a hand mixer until frothy.

2. Add almonds then toss until everything sticks. Transfer the almonds to the slow cooker.
3. Add everything else except water and toss.
4. Cook for about 3 hours on low stirring often.
5. Add water, mix and cook for an additional 30 minutes.
6. Transfer to a parchment paper to cool and harden.
7. Serve and enjoy.

NUTRITION: Calories: 219, total fat: 19g, saturated fat: 13g, total carbs: 6g, net carbs: 2g, protein: 6g, sugars: 3g, fiber: 4g, sodium: 698mg, potassium: 412mg

101. Chocolate Chip Cookies

Prep time: 20 minutes

Cooking Time: 4 hours

Servings: 12

INGREDIENTS

- 2 eggs, organic
- ½ cup coconut oil, room temperature
- 2 tbsp vanilla
- ½ cup stevia
- 1½ cup chia, gluten-free
- ½ cup flax, ground
- ½ tbsp baking powder
- ½ tbsp salt
- ¾ cup dark chocolate chips, sugar-free

DIRECTIONS:

1. Grease your slow cooker bottom with oil then fit a piece of wax paper to the bottom. Grease the wax paper with oil too.
2. Mix eggs, coconut oil, vanilla and stevia in a medium bowl.
3. Add the rest of the ingredients except chips in another separate bowl and mix to combine well.
4. Mix the dry ingredients with wet ingredients then stir in chocolate chips until combined.
5. Place and spread the dough into the slow cooker insert then make the top smooth.
6. Cook for about 2½ - 3 hours on low until a set center. When a toothpick is placed in the center, it should come out clean.

7. Remove the insert and cool for about 30 minutes then transfer the wax paper with dough on a wire rack to cool for an additional 30 minutes.

8. Cut into bars when cooled completely.

9. Serve immediately. You can store in a container, airtight, for about 3-5 days.

NUTRITION: Calories: 224, total Fat: 15.2g, saturated fat: 10.5g, total carbs: 17.6g, net carbs: 14.3g, protein: 4.2g, sugars: 14g, fiber: 3.3g, sodium: 131mg, potassium: 102mg

30-DAY MEAL PLAN

DAY	BREAKFAST	MAIN DISH	SIDE DISH	DESSERT
1	Apple and Onion Omelet	Slow-Cooked Lemon Chicken	Roasted Garlic White Bean Dip	Blackberry Mountain Pie
2	Avocado Toast with Egg	Chunky Beef and Potato Slow Roast	Crab and Carrot Dip	Lemon Squares
3	Baked Egg Cups	Lemony Haddock	Roasted Garlic White Bean Dip	Baked Apple Pie
4	Apple and Cinnamon French Toast Strata	Curry Chicken	Roasted Garlic White Bean Dip	Homemade applesauce
5	Grilled Veggie and Cheese Bagel	Sticky Pulled Beef Open Sandwiches	Green Goddess Dip	Whipped Strawberry Mousse
6	Baked Egg Cups	Turkey Sausages	Crab and Carrot Dip	Scarlet's Frozen Fantasy
7	Chorizo and Egg Tortilla	Oregano Salmon with Crunchy Crust	Roasted Mint Carrots	Ribbon Cakes
8	Grilled Veggie and Cheese Bagel	Spicy Lamb	Roasted Garlic White Bean Dip	Lemon Squares
9	Avocado Toast with Egg	Roasted Citrus Chicken	Roasted Garlic White Bean Dip	Baked Egg Custard
10	Grilled Veggie and Cheese Bagel	Tuna Casserole	Roasted Mint Carrots	Baked Apple Pie
11	Chorizo and Egg Tortilla	Herby Beef Stroganoff and Fluffy Rice	Roasted Root Vegetables	Jeweled Cookies
12	Apple and Onion Omelet	Spiced Lamb Burgers	Roasted Garlic White Bean Dip	Lemon Squares
13	Grilled Veggie and Cheese Bagel	Slow-Cooked Bavarian Pot Roast	Roasted Root Vegetables	Scarlet's Frozen Fantasy
14	Grilled Veggie and Cheese Bagel	Glazed Salmon	Green Goddess Dip	Ribbon Cakes
15	Apple and Cinnamon French Toast Strata	Chunky Beef and Potato Slow Roast	Roasted Garlic White Bean Dip	Baked Egg Custard
16	Asparagus and Cauliflower Tortilla	Chicken Adobo	Roasted Garlic White Bean Dip	Creamy Pineapple Dessert
17	Breakfast Casserole	Chicken with Asian Vegetables	Roasted Root Vegetables	Whipped Strawberry Mousse
18	Avocado Toast with Egg	Poached Gennaro/Sea Bass with Red Peppers	Green Goddess Dip	Homemade applesauce

19	Breakfast Casserole	Aromatic Chicken and Cabbage Stir-Fry	Vegetable Couscous	Baked Apple Pie
20	Asparagus and Cauliflower Tortilla	Mouthwatering Beef and Chilli Stew	Vegetable Couscous	Ice cream sandwiches
21	Chorizo and Egg Tortilla	Shrimp Skewers with Mango Cucumber Salsa	Roasted Mint Carrots	Pineapple Pudding
22	Avocado Toast with Egg	Beef One-Pot Slow Roast	Crab and Carrot Dip	Baked Egg Custard
23	Apple and Onion Omelet	Sardine Fish Cakes	Roasted Root Vegetables	Pineapple Pudding
24	Asparagus and Cauliflower Tortilla	Chicken Adobo	Green Goddess Dip	Ice cream sandwiches
25	Apple and Onion Omelet	Classic Beef Stroganoff with Egg Noodles	Crab and Carrot Dip	Jeweled Cookies
26	Apple and Cinnamon French Toast Strata	Pineapple and Mint Lamb Chops	Roasted Root Vegetables	Whipped Strawberry Mousse
27	Avocado Toast with Egg	Slow-Cooked Bavarian Pot Roast	Roasted Mint Carrots	Pineapple Pudding
28	Apple and Onion Omelet	Beef and Three Pepper Stew	Vegetable Couscous	Creamy Pineapple Dessert
29	Baked Egg Cups	Cajun Catfish	Crab and Carrot Dip	Scarlet's Frozen Fantasy
30	Avocado Toast with Egg	Roast Pork Loin with Sweet and Tart Apple Stuffing	Vegetable Couscous	Blackberry Mountain P

CONCLUSION

Thanks for making it to the end of the renal diet cookbook. Renal diet is one of the most challenging diets to follow, and because of its limited choice, the temptation to stray from it is high. This is why meals need to be made with special care, so that they don't disappoint. Every meal must be planned to be as rich in nutrients as possible. This is the reason why we compiled this cookbook for you. We hope you find these recipes as simple to prepare as they are delicious to eat.

You can count on us to bring you the most delicious renal diet cookbook. Our dietitians and chefs have designed a variety of tasty recipes for your convenience. The renal diet is a rich source of proteins, complex carbohydrates, and fibers, and along with it being low on sodium and fat, it is undoubtedly the healthiest diet. We are here to make it easy for you. You don't have to worry about your family or friends being deprived of great food while you are on this diet.

Our recipes are designed for you to please everyone who loves food, and you will surely enjoy them too!